RABBIT CARE ESSENTIALS

A Guide to Raising Happy Bunnies

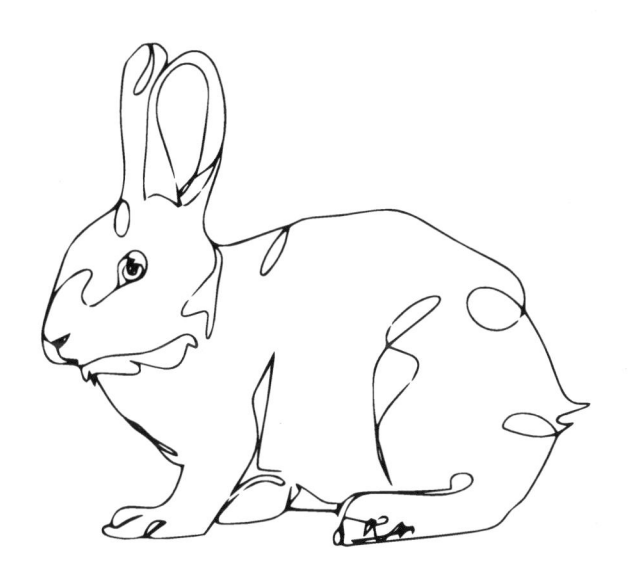

Ryan Warner

Copyright © 2024 Ryan Warner
All Rights Reserved.

Contents

Introduction	**2**
Misconceptions to Owning Rabbits	3
CHAPTER 1	
Understanding Your Rabbit	**6**
Introduction to Rabbit Breeds	7
Popular Pet Rabbit Breeds and Their Characteristics	8
Rabbit Behavior and Social Needs	15
Understanding Rabbit Instincts and Socialization	16
Importance of Companionship and Play	16
Understanding Rabbit Instincts	18
CHAPTER 2	
Finding Your Perfect Rabbit	**20**
What Should I Look for in a Rabbit?	21
What Breeds Make Good Pets?	22
Where Can I Buy/Adopt a Rabbit?	24
What Should I Do to Check the Health and Wellness of a Rabbit Before Bringing Them Home?	25
CHAPTER 3	
Setting Up a Rabbit-Friendly Home	**28**
Creating the Ideal Living Space	29
Cage vs. Free-Range Living: Pros and Cons	29
Essential Supplies: Bedding, Hiding Spots, and Toys	32

Safety Considerations	33
Rabbit-proofing your home and garden	33
Identifying Toxic Plants and Hazards	35
Additional Considerations for a Rabbit-Friendly Home	36

CHAPTER 4
Nutrition Essentials for Your Rabbit — 38

Understanding a Rabbit's Dietary Needs	39
Importance of Hay, Fresh Vegetables, and Pellets	39
Safe and Unsafe Foods for Rabbits	41
Supplements for Optimal Health	43
Overview of Vitamins and Minerals	43
When and How to Use Supplements	43
Additional Nutritional Considerations	45

CHAPTER 5
Litter Box Training Your Rabbit — 48

The Basics of Litter Box Training	49
Choosing the Right Litter & Box Size	49
Steps to Successfully Train Your Rabbit	50
Common Challenges and Solutions	51
Troubleshooting Accidents	52
Behavioral Issues	53
Additional Tips for Successful Litter Box Training	54
Detailed Examination of Behavioral Issues	55
Maintaining a Healthy Litter Box Environment	56
Encouraging Positive Behavior	57

CHAPTER 6
Health and Wellness — 60

Routine Veterinary Care	61

Importance of Spaying/Neutering and Vaccinations   61
Recognizing signs of illness in rabbits   63
Preventative Health Measures: 67
   Grooming   67
   Dental Care   69
   Maintaining a Healthy Weight   70

CHAPTER 7
Understanding Rabbit Behavior and Training Techniques   74

Basic Commands and Tricks   75
   Teaching Your Rabbit to Come, Stay, and Other Simple Commands   75
Addressing Behavioral Issues   77
   Solutions for Common Problems like Chewing and Digging   77
   Advanced Training Techniques   80
   Dealing with Fearful or Timid Rabbits   81
   Socialization and Bonding   82
   Addressing Specific Behavioral Issues   83

CHAPTER 8
Enrichment and Exercise   86

The Importance of Mental and Physical Stimulation and Understanding Rabbit Behavior   87
   Ideas for Interactive Toys and Activities   87
Creating a Playtime Routine   89
   Importance of a Structured Routine   89
   Safe Outdoor Play   90
   Bonding Activities   91
   Advanced Enrichment Ideas   92
   The Benefits of Socialization   94
   Environmental Design for Rabbit Well-Being   94
   Routine and Consistency   95

CHAPTER 9
Fun Tips for Rabbit Owners   98

    Creative Ways to Interact and Bond with Your Rabbit   99

Celebrating Special Occasions with Your Rabbit   102

    Ideas for Rabbit-Themed Parties and Events   102

Community and Resources   104

    Connecting with Other Rabbit Owners and Finding Support   104

Closing Notes from the Author   108

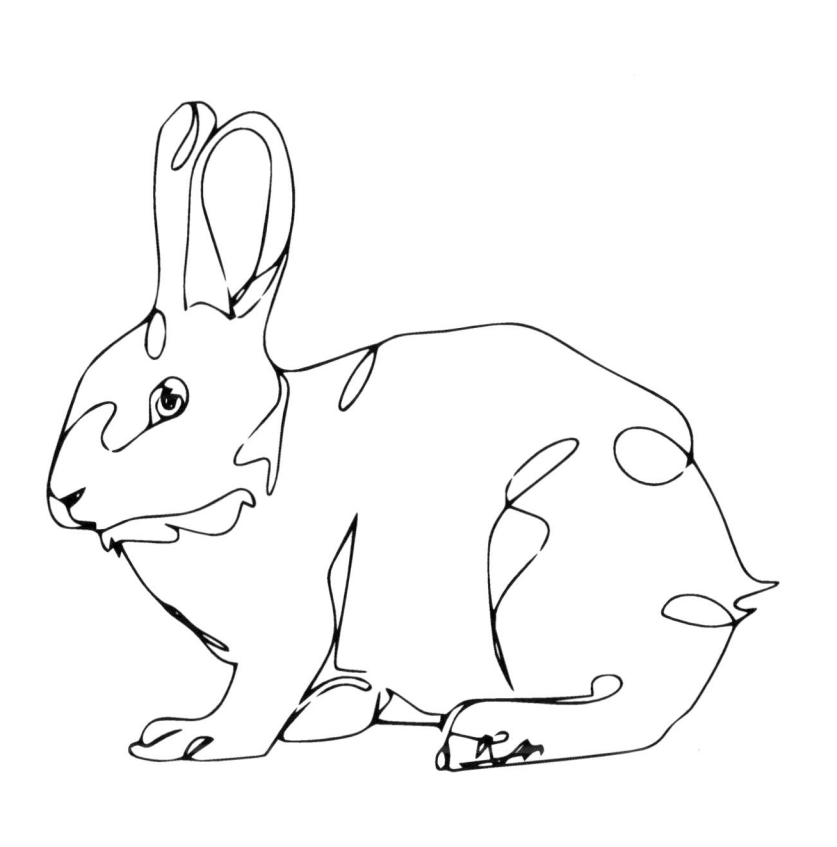

INTRODUCTION

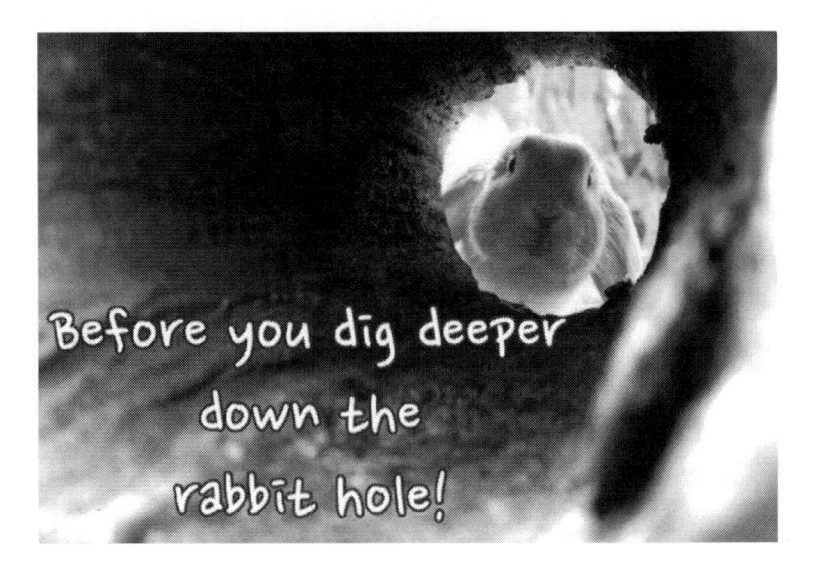

Before you dig deeper down the rabbit hole!

Congratulations on discovering this comprehensive guide to rabbit care, built on decades of experience in successfully hand-raising rabbits. It is our hope that you are exploring this material before embarking on the journey of rabbit ownership, which can be both rewarding and complex.

This manual aims to enhance your understanding and appreciation of these remarkable animals. It is important to recognize that not all rabbits are the same; some are better suited for companionship while others may be more appropriate for culinary purposes. However, this book will focus exclusively on the aspects of rabbit ownership related to companionship.

By the time you reach the midpoint of this book, you will have gained insights into different rabbit breeds and their suitability for you and your family. Key considerations such as size, temperament, and special care requirements will be discussed to help you make informed decisions before welcoming a new furry family member into your home.

Drawing upon over 25 years of expertise in rabbit care, this all-encompassing guide covers essential responsibilities, best practices, and common pitfalls. If you are passionate about rabbits and considering ownership, this book is designed to steer you in the right direction. Our goal is to empower you to provide the best possible life for your rabbit, making this book your trusted resource in the journey ahead. We will address vital topics that contribute to the health, happiness, and longevity of your pet rabbit.

Misconceptions to Owning Rabbits

The average person thinks "Rabbits are Easy!". There are several common misconceptions about rabbit care that can lead to misunderstandings and inadequate treatment of these animals.

Here are some of the most prevalent ones:

1. **Rabbits Are Low-Maintenance Pets:** Many people believe rabbits require little care, but they need daily attention, social interaction, and specific dietary needs.
2. **Rabbits Can Live on Carrots:** While carrots are often associated with rabbits, they should only be an occasional treat. A proper diet consists mainly of hay, fresh vegetables, and specially formulated pellets.
3. **Rabbits Are Just Like Cats or Dogs:** Rabbits have different social needs and behaviors compared to cats and dogs. They require specific training, socialization, and care that cater to their unique instincts.

4. **Rabbits Don't Need Exercise:** Some believe that rabbits can stay in their cage all day. However, they need ample space to run, hop, and play outside of their cage to maintain health and prevent obesity.
5. **It's Okay to Keep a Single Rabbit:** Rabbits are social animals and thrive in the company of their kind. While they can bond with humans, having a companion rabbit is often better for their mental health, especially female rabbits.
6. **Litter Training is Impossible:** Many people think rabbits cannot be litter trained. In reality, with patience and the right techniques, most rabbits can learn to use a litter box effectively. Stay tuned, we go in-depth on this later in the book.
7. **Rabbits Don't Need Veterinary Care:** Some rabbit owners underestimate the importance of regular veterinary check-ups. Rabbits require routine health care, including vaccinations and dental checks.
8. **Rabbits Don't Show Affection:** While rabbits may not express affection in the same way as dogs, they can form strong bonds with their owners and show affection through grooming, nudging, and cuddling.
9. **All Rabbits Can Be Free-Roaming:** Not all rabbits are suitable for free-roaming environments. Some may need more supervision than others, depending on their temperament and safety concerns in the home.
10. **Rabbits Are Quiet Pets:** While rabbits are generally quieter than dogs, they can make various sounds and may thump or grunt as a way to communicate or express discomfort.

Understanding these misconceptions can help potential rabbit owners provide better care and create a more enriching environment for their pets.

CHAPTER 1
UNDERSTANDING YOUR RABBIT

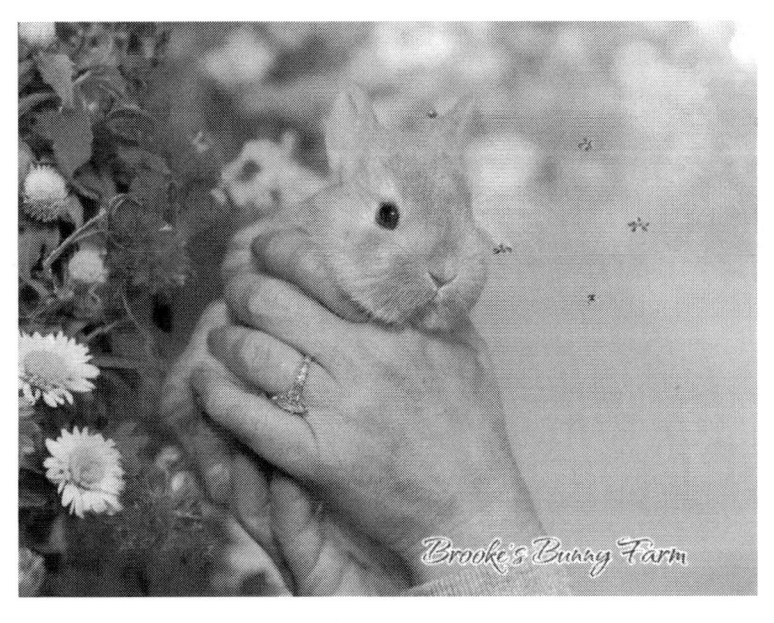

(Picture of Baby Netherland Dwarf courtesy of Brooke's Bunny Farm, CT)

Rabbits are a diverse group of animals, with more than 50 recognized breeds ranging in size, temperament, and care needs. Choosing the right breed is crucial for a positive and fulfilling pet ownership experience.

Rabbits are fascinating and gentle creatures, each with its own unique personality and characteristics. To ensure that your rabbit thrives in its environment, it is important to understand the various rabbit breeds, their behaviors, and social needs. This chapter will delve into popular rabbit breeds and their traits, as well as the instincts that define rabbit behavior and the importance of socialization and companionship.

Introduction to Rabbit Breeds

Rabbits come in various breeds, each offering distinct characteristics. Understanding these breeds can help potential rabbit owners choose the right pet that fits their lifestyle. When selecting a breed, consider the rabbit's size, activity level, grooming requirements, and temperament to ensure it aligns with your lifestyle and space availability.

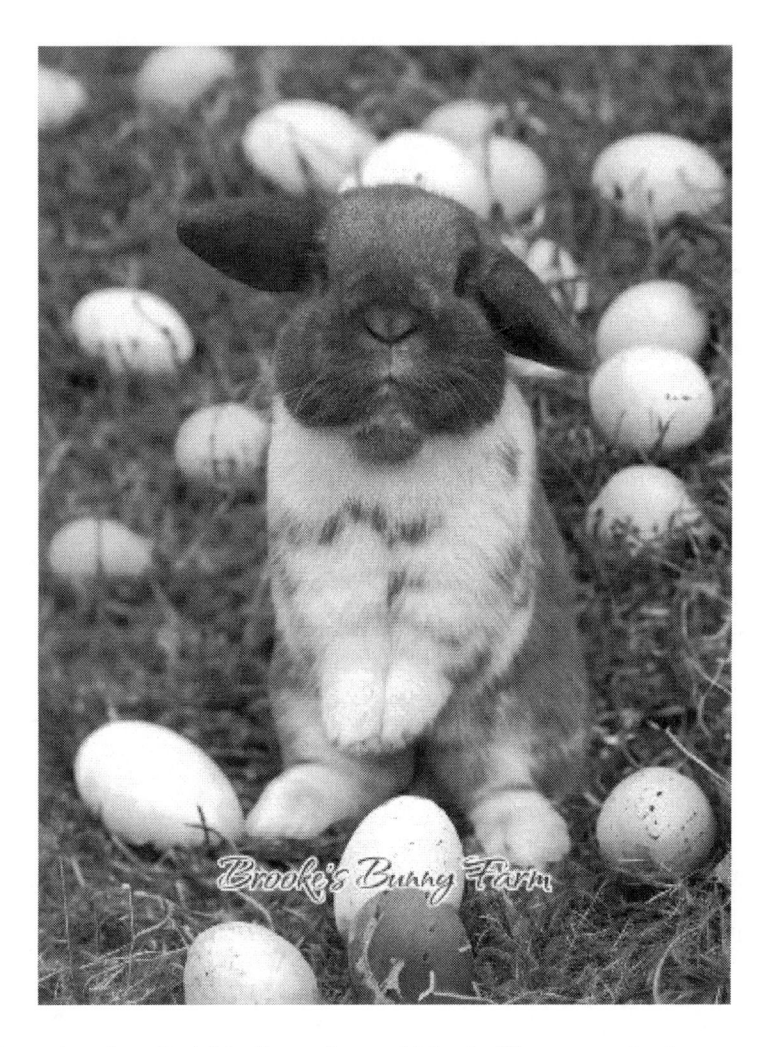

Popular Pet Rabbit Breeds and Their Characteristics

1. Holland Lop:

Size: Small (2-4 lbs.)
Temperament: Friendly and affectionate
Characteristics: Known for their floppy ears and compact body, Holland Lops are playful and enjoy interaction. They are excellent pets for families and individuals alike.

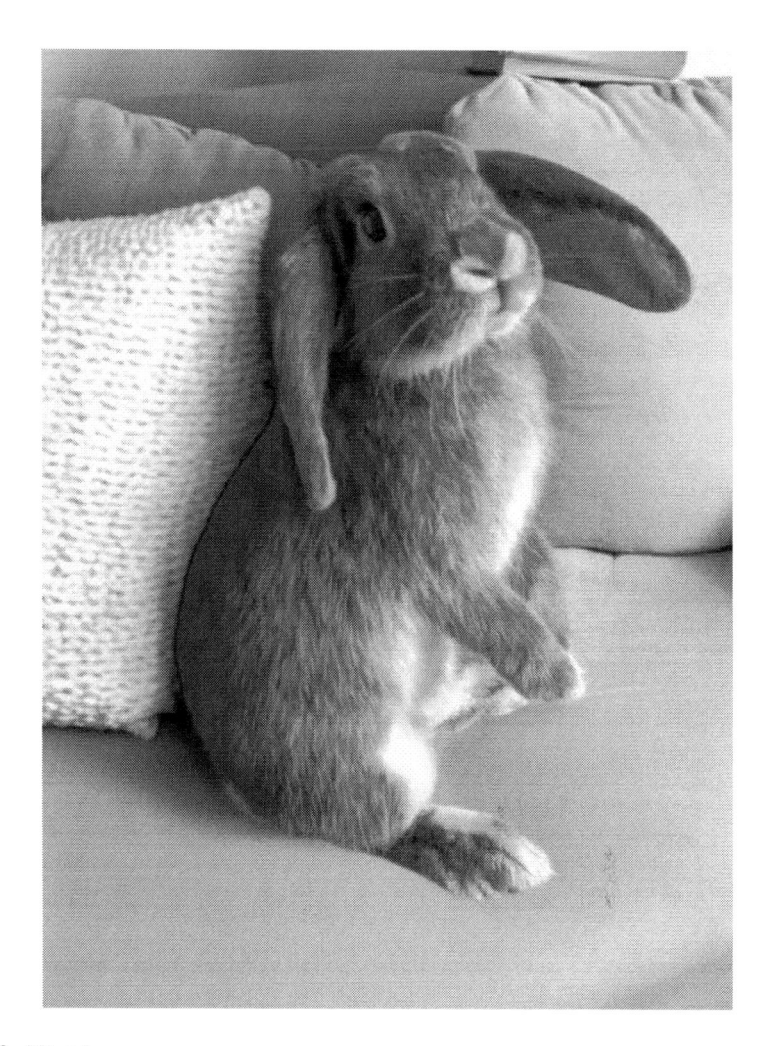

2. Mini Lop:

Size: Small to medium (4-6 lbs.)

Temperament: Friendly, affectionate, and playful.

Characteristics: This breed is larger than the Holland Lop but still yields a compact body with lop ears that hang down. This breed requires regular grooming, especially during shedding seasons.

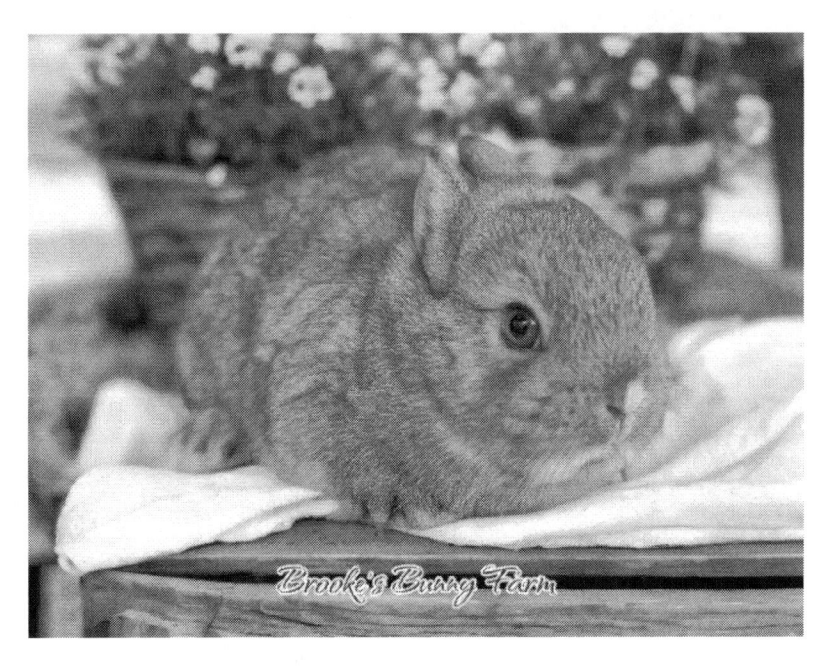

3. Netherland Dwarf:

Size: Very small (1.5-3 lbs.)

Temperament: Energetic and curious

Characteristics: This breed is one of the smallest and is known for its round face and small size. They are highly energetic and enjoy exploring their surroundings.

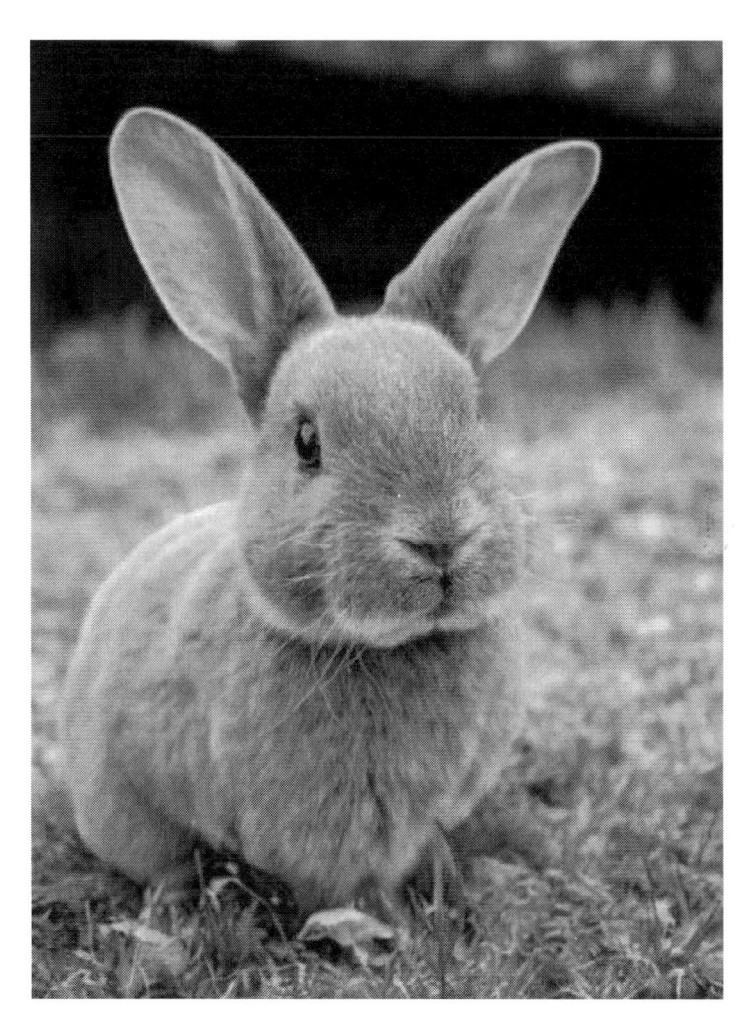

4. Mini Rex:

Size: Small to medium (3-4.5 lbs.)
Temperament: Gentle and calm
Characteristics: Recognized for their velvety fur, Mini Rex rabbits are easy to handle and often enjoy being held. They have a friendly disposition and adapt well to families.

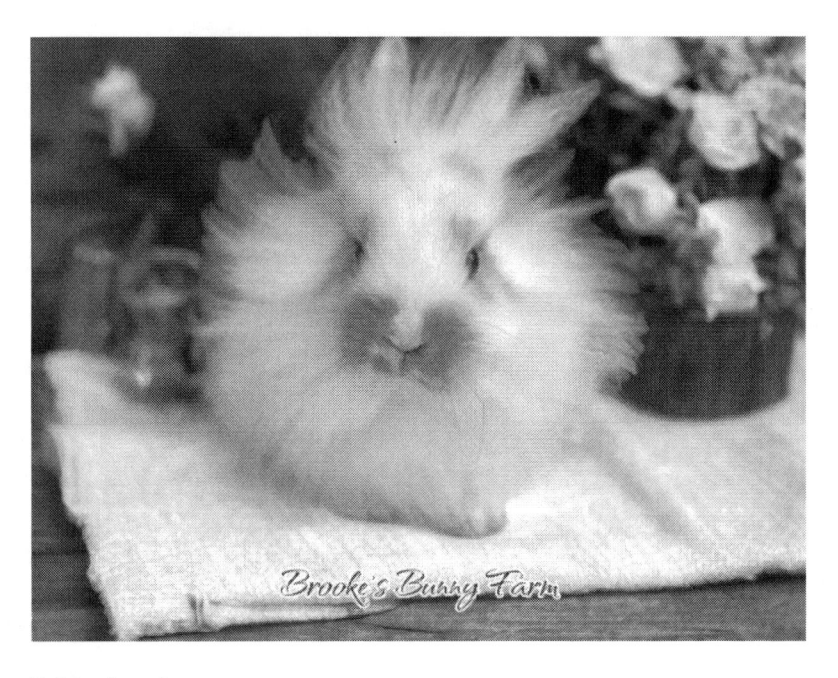

5. Lionhead:

Size: Small (3-5 lbs.)

Temperament: Social and playful

Characteristics: The Lionhead breed is distinguished by its mane of fur around the head. They are known for their playful nature and enjoy engaging with their owners.

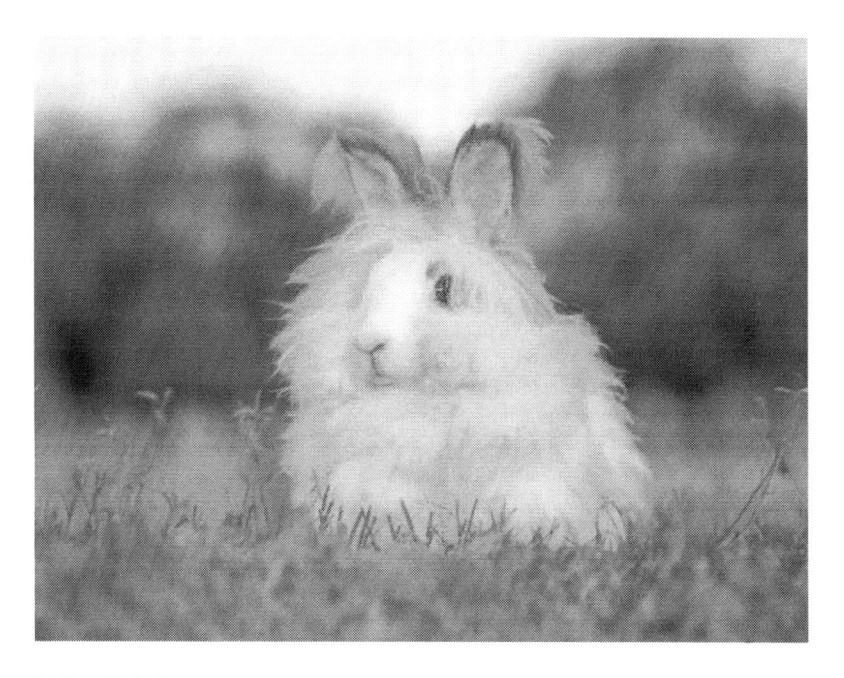

6. English Angora:

Size: Medium (5.5-7.5 lbs.)

Temperament: Gentle and affectionate

Characteristics: With their long, fluffy fur, English Angoras require regular grooming. They are calm and enjoy being petted, making them great companions.

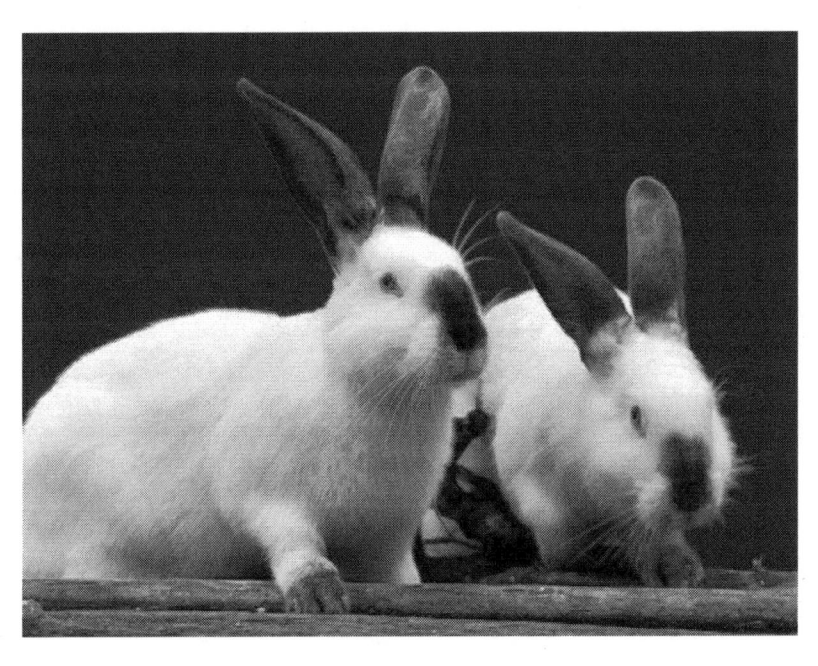

7. California Rabbit:

Size: Large (8-12 lbs.)

Temperament: Friendly and docile

Characteristics: This breed is known for its distinctive white fur with black markings. They have an easygoing nature, making them suitable for families.

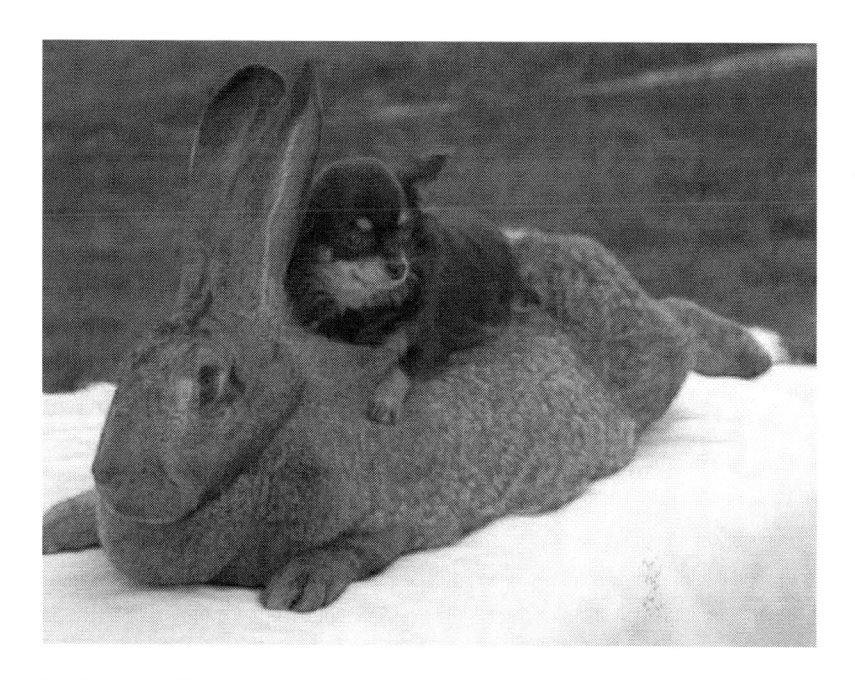

8. Flemish Giant:

Size: Very large (14-20 lbs.)

Temperament: Gentle and friendly

Characteristics: As one of the largest rabbit breeds, Flemish Giants are known for their calm demeanor. They enjoy being around people and require ample space to move.

Understanding these breeds helps prospective owners choose a rabbit that matches their lifestyle and expectations. Each breed has its unique needs, and compatibility with the owner's environment is crucial for a happy pet.

Rabbit Behavior and Social Needs

Rabbits are complex creatures with specific instincts and social behaviors. Understanding these can enhance the bond between the owner and the rabbit, leading to a fulfilling relationship.

Understanding Rabbit Instincts and Socialization

Rabbits are prey animals, and their instincts are rooted in survival. This means they are naturally cautious and may exhibit behaviors such as thumping, hiding, or freezing when they feel threatened. Recognizing these instincts is essential for understanding rabbit behavior and ensuring their comfort.

1. **Thumping:** When a rabbit thumps its hind leg, it is signaling danger or alerting others. This behavior is an instinctual response to potential threats.
2. **Hiding:** Rabbits often seek out hiding spots when they feel insecure or scared. Providing safe, cozy spaces in their habitat can help them feel more secure.
3. **Grooming:** Grooming is a social behavior among rabbits. They groom themselves and may also groom their owners or other rabbits, which is a sign of affection and bonding.
4. **Exploration:** Rabbits are naturally curious and enjoy exploring their environment. Allowing them supervised time outside their cage can satisfy their curiosity and provide mental stimulation.

Importance of Companionship and Play

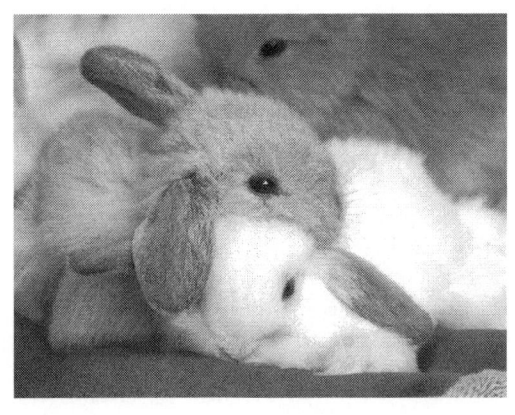

Rabbits thrive on companionship. In the wild, they live in groups, and isolation can lead to boredom and depression. If possible, consider adopting a bonded pair or investing significant time in socializing with your rabbit daily.

Socialization is critical for a rabbit's well-being. As social animals, rabbits thrive in the company of other rabbits or pets. Here are some key points regarding companionship and play:

1. Companionship

Rabbits are happiest when they have a companion. Having another rabbit or even a compatible pet can reduce loneliness and encourage social behaviors, such as grooming and playing together. If considering a second rabbit, ensure they are properly introduced to prevent territorial disputes.

2. Playtime

Regular playtime is essential for a rabbit's physical and mental health. Engaging with toys, tunnels, and interactive games can keep a rabbit entertained and prevent boredom. Daily play sessions also strengthen the bond between the rabbit and its owner.

Physical and mental stimulation are vital. Rabbits need at least 3-4 hours of supervised playtime outside their enclosure daily. Provide toys, tunnels, and space to hop, which supports their physical health and prevents destructive behaviors.

3. Routine Interaction

Rabbits enjoy interacting with their owners through gentle petting, feeding, or play. Building trust takes time, especially with timid rabbits, but patience and consistency are key.

Spending quality time with your rabbit is crucial. Regular petting, gentle handling, and interactive play help build trust and strengthen the relationship. Rabbits can recognize their owners and respond positively to affection.

4. Behavioral Enrichment

Providing opportunities for mental stimulation, such as puzzle toys or treat-dispensing devices, can enhance your rabbit's environment. This prevents destructive behaviors that may arise from boredom.

5. Bonding with Other Rabbits:

Bonding two rabbits requires a gradual introduction in a neutral space. Look for signs of compatibility, such as grooming each other, and avoid placing rabbits together if there's aggression like biting or lunging.

Meeting your rabbit's social and behavioral needs is the foundation of a happy, healthy life. A well-socialized rabbit is more affectionate, confident, and likely to develop a strong bond with its owner.

To care for a rabbit properly, it's essential to understand their natural behavior and social requirements. Rabbits are prey animals with unique instincts and a strong need for companionship and mental stimulation.

Understanding Rabbit Instincts

Prey Instincts

Rabbits are naturally cautious. Quick movements, loud noises, or unfamiliar environments can make them nervous. They communicate fear through body language, such as thumping their hind legs or freezing in place.

Foraging and Digging

Wild rabbits forage for food and dig burrows, instincts that remain strong in domesticated rabbits. Providing hay, chew toys, and digging boxes can help satisfy these natural behaviors.

Territorial Behavior

Rabbits may mark their territory with chin rubs (scent glands on their chin) or droppings. Depending on breed, spaying or neutering can reduce territorial aggression and improves social behavior with humans, rabbits or other family pets.

Curiosity

Rabbits are intelligent and inquisitive animals that enjoy exploring their surroundings. Rabbit-proof your home to prevent accidents, as they love chewing cords, furniture, or other household items.

Chapter Summary

This section of the chapter lays the groundwork for understanding your rabbit's unique needs and personality, ensuring a harmonious and rewarding relationship with your new pet. Understanding your rabbit involves recognizing the various breeds and their specific characteristics, as well as grasping the social and behavioral needs of these animals. By providing the right environment, companionship, and engaging activities, you can ensure that your rabbit leads a happy, healthy, and fulfilling life.

CHAPTER 2
FINDING YOUR PERFECT RABBIT

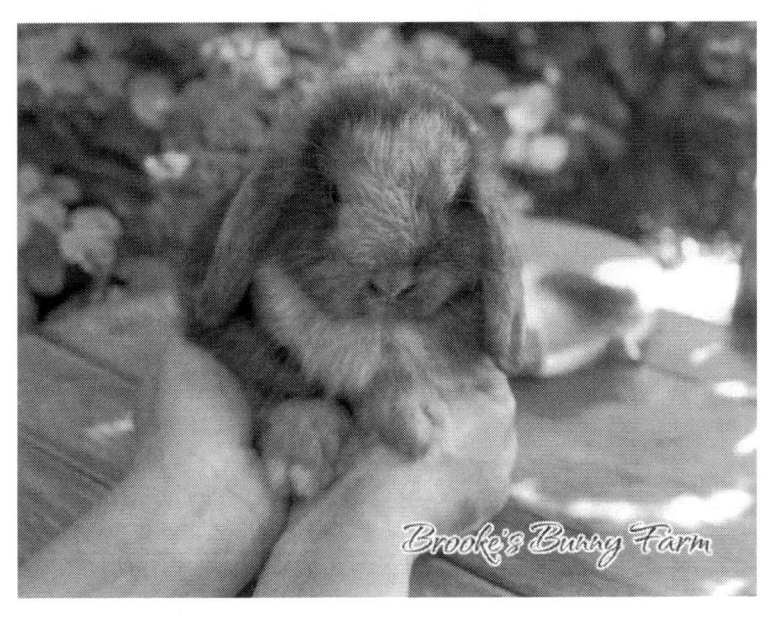

(Picture of Baby Holland Lop courtesy of Brooke's Bunny Farm, CT)

Choosing the right rabbit to bring into your home is a significant decision that requires careful consideration. This chapter will guide you through the essential factors to consider when selecting a rabbit, highlight breeds that make excellent pets, provide information on where to adopt or buy a rabbit, and outline the health and wellness checks you should perform before bringing a rabbit home.

What Should I Look for in a Rabbit?

When selecting a rabbit, there are several key factors to consider to ensure that you find a good match for your lifestyle and preferences:

1. Personality and Temperament:

- Different rabbits exhibit varying temperaments. Some may be more social and outgoing, while others might be shy and reserved. Spend time interacting with potential rabbits to gauge their behavior and see how they respond to handling and attention.
- Look for a rabbit that appears curious and engages with you. A friendly rabbit will approach you, allow you to pet them, and show signs of comfort and trust.

2. Age:

- Rabbits can be adopted at different ages, from young kits to adult rabbits. Younger rabbits may require more training and socialization, while older rabbits may already have established personalities.
- Consider your lifestyle when choosing the age of your rabbit. If you have the time and patience to train a young rabbit, a kit may be a good choice. If you prefer a rabbit with a more predictable temperament, an adult rabbit might be ideal.

3. Energy Level:

- Rabbits have different energy levels, with some being more active and playful, while others are more laid-back. Assess your own energy level and how much time you can dedicate to play and interaction.
- An active rabbit may require more space and toys for enrichment, while a calmer rabbit may be content with less stimulation.

4. Size:

- Rabbits come in various sizes, from small breeds like the Holland Lop to larger breeds like the Flemish Giant. Consider your living space and the size of the rabbit when making your decision.
- Larger rabbits may require more room to move around and may need larger supplies, while smaller rabbits can thrive in more confined spaces.

5. Grooming Needs:

- Different breeds have varying grooming requirements. Long-haired breeds, such as Angoras, require regular grooming to prevent matting, while short-haired breeds may need less maintenance.
- Assess your willingness and ability to commit time to grooming based on the rabbit's coat type.

What Breeds Make Good Pets?

Several rabbit breeds are known for their friendly and sociable nature, making them excellent pets. Here are a few popular breeds to consider:

1. Holland Lop:

Characteristics: Small, friendly, and affectionate, Holland Lops are known for their gentle temperament and playful nature.

Grooming: Low grooming needs, but regular brushing is recommended to prevent matting.

2. Netherland Dwarf:

Characteristics: Compact and energetic, Netherland Dwarfs are curious and social, often forming strong bonds with their owners.

Grooming: Low grooming needs, but they benefit from regular handling to maintain their social nature.

3. Mini Rex:

Characteristics: Known for their soft, velvety coats and friendly demeanor, Mini Rex rabbits are playful and enjoy being handled.

Grooming: Minimal grooming required, making them relatively low-maintenance.

4. Lionhead:

Characteristics: Recognizable by their fluffy manes, Lionheads are friendly and inquisitive, often enjoying human interaction.

Grooming: Moderate grooming needs due to their long fur; regular brushing is necessary.

5. English Angora:

Characteristics: Known for their long, luxurious fur, English Angoras are gentle and affectionate, making them great companions.

Grooming: High grooming needs, requiring regular brushing to prevent matting and keep their fur healthy.

6. Flemish Giant:

Characteristics: One of the largest rabbit breeds, Flemish Giants are known for their calm and gentle nature. They are often referred to as "gentle giants."

Grooming: Low grooming needs, but they require ample space due to their size.

Where Can I Buy/Adopt a Rabbit?

When it comes to finding a rabbit, you have several options to consider:

1. Animal Shelters and Rescues:

- Adopting from a shelter or rescue not only provides a home to a rabbit in need but also helps reduce the number of homeless pets. Many shelters have rabbits of various breeds and ages available for adoption.
- Look for local animal shelters or rabbit-specific rescues in your area. Websites like Petfinder and Adopt-a-Pet can help you locate rabbits available for adoption.

2. Reputable Breeders:

- If you choose to purchase a rabbit, ensure that you find a reputable breeder who prioritizes the health and well-being of their rabbits. A good breeder will provide a clean and safe environment, socialization for their rabbits, and health records.

- Ask for references, visit the breeder's facility, and observe the conditions in which the rabbits are raised. Responsible breeders will be knowledgeable about their breeds and be willing to answer your questions.

3. Pet Stores:

- While some pet stores offer rabbits for sale, it is essential to do thorough research before purchasing from a store. Many pet store rabbits come from commercial breeding operations that may not prioritize health and socialization.
- If you opt to buy from a pet store, ensure the store provides proper care and health guarantees, and be prepared to take on any necessary socialization and training.

What Should I Do to Check the Health and Wellness of a Rabbit Before Bringing Them Home?

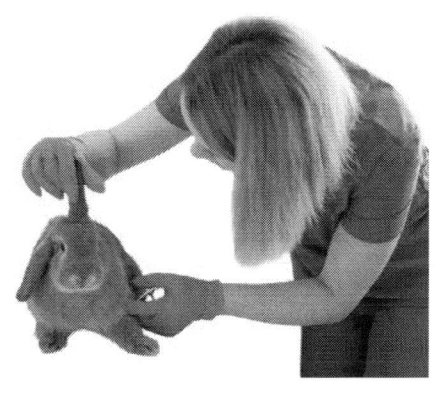

Before bringing a rabbit home, it is crucial to assess their health and wellness to ensure you are adopting a healthy pet. Here are steps to take when checking a rabbit's health:

1. Physical Examination:

Eyes and Ears: Check for clear eyes without discharge and clean, upright ears. Redness or discharge can indicate health issues.

Nose and Mouth: Look for a clean nose without discharge and healthy gums and teeth. Teeth should be aligned and not overgrown.

Fur and Skin: Examine the coat for any signs of matting, bald spots, or parasites. Healthy rabbits have clean, shiny fur.

Body Condition: Gently palpate the rabbit's body to check for a healthy weight. You should feel their ribs without excessive fat covering.

2. Behavioral Observations:

- Observe the rabbit's behavior in its current environment. A healthy rabbit will be alert, curious, and active. Look for signs of lethargy or hiding, which can indicate stress or illness.
- Pay attention to how the rabbit interacts with people and other rabbits. A friendly, social rabbit is more likely to adapt well to a new home.

3. Ask About Health History:

- Inquire about the rabbit's health history, including any vaccinations, spaying/neutering, and previous medical issues. A reputable seller or rescue should be able to provide you with health records.
- If adopting from a shelter, ask about any known behavioral issues or special needs the rabbit may have.

4. Veterinary Check-Up:

- Before bringing your rabbit home, consider scheduling a veterinary check-up to ensure they are in good health. A veterinarian who specializes in rabbit care can perform a thorough examination and provide valuable advice on care.
- Discuss vaccinations, diet, and any specific health concerns with the veterinarian to set a solid foundation for your rabbit's well-being.

Chapter Summary

Finding the perfect rabbit for your home is an exciting journey that requires thoughtful consideration of various factors, including personality, breed characteristics, and health. By understanding what to look for in a rabbit, exploring suitable breeds, and knowing where to adopt or buy, you can make an informed decision that aligns with your lifestyle.

Conducting thorough health checks before bringing a rabbit home is crucial to ensuring a smooth transition and a healthy start to your relationship. With the right preparation and understanding, you can find a loving companion that will enrich your life for years to come. As you embark on this rewarding journey, remember that each rabbit is unique, and building a strong bond will take time, patience, and love.

CHAPTER 3
SETTING UP A RABBIT-FRIENDLY HOME

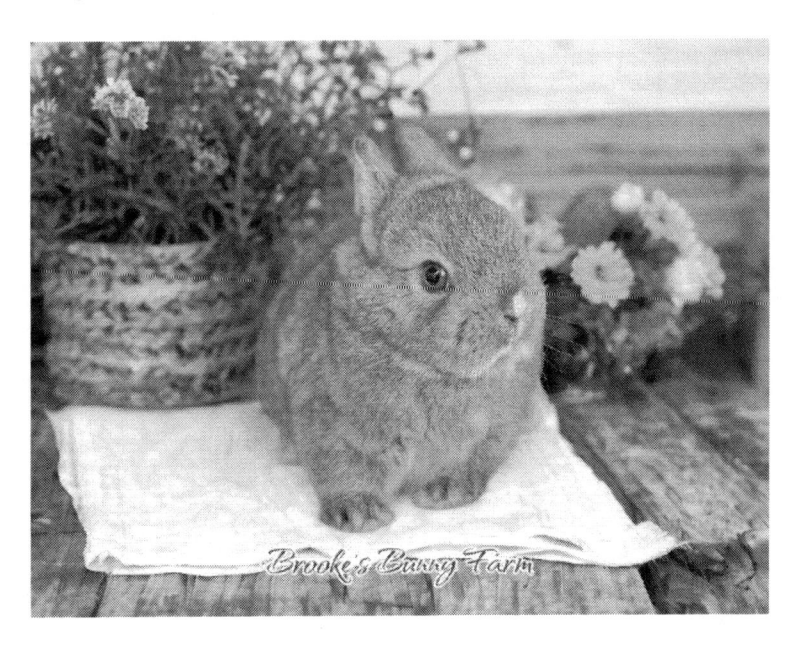

Creating a comfortable and safe environment for your rabbit is essential for its well-being. This chapter will guide you through setting up the ideal living space for your furry friend, discussing the pros and cons of different living arrangements, essential supplies needed for their care, and crucial safety considerations to protect your rabbit from potential hazards.

Creating the Ideal Living Space

When it comes to housing your rabbit, there are two primary options: cages and free-range living. Each has its benefits and drawbacks, and understanding these can help you decide what is best for your pet.

Cage vs. Free-Range Living: Pros and Cons
Cage Living
Pros:

- **Controlled Environment:** A cage provides a safe and confined space for your rabbit, minimizing the risk of accidents or injuries.
- **Easy Cleanup:** Maintaining a clean area is simpler when using a designated cage, making it easier to manage waste and litter.
- **Security:** A cage can protect your rabbit from other pets, children, and environmental dangers when you cannot supervise them.

Cons:

- **Limited Space:** Spending too much time in a cage can lead to boredom and stress for your rabbit. It is essential to ensure they have ample time outside the cage for exercise and exploration.

- **Less Interaction:** A cage may limit your rabbit's social interactions, which can affect their mental well-being if they are not given enough attention.

Cage Size: When choosing a cage, size matters. The cage should be large enough for your rabbit to stand up on its hind legs, turn around comfortably, and lie down fully stretched out. A good rule of thumb is to have a cage that is at least four times the size of your rabbit.

Multi-Level Cages: Consider multi-level cages that provide vertical space for climbing and exploring. This can help simulate a more natural environment and allow for more movement.

Free-Range Living

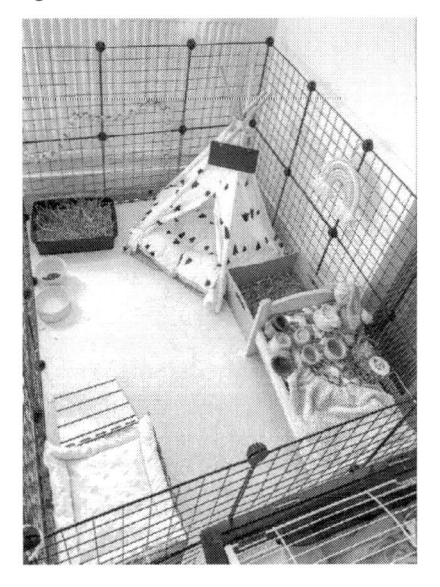

Pros:

- **Enhanced Freedom:** Free-range living allows your rabbit to explore and roam, promoting natural behaviors such as hopping, digging, and foraging.

- **Socialization:** Being out and about provides more opportunities for interaction with family members, enhancing the bond between you and your rabbit.
- **Physical Activity:** More space encourages exercise, helping to maintain a healthy weight and prevent obesity.

Cons:

- **Potential Hazards:** Free-range rabbits may encounter dangers such as toxic plants, electrical cords, or small objects that can be ingested.
- **Supervision Required:** You must supervise your rabbit during free-range time to prevent accidents and ensure their safety.
- **Increased Cleanup:** A larger area can lead to more mess, making it essential to regularly clean up droppings and debris.

Designated Play Area: If you opt for free-range living, consider creating a designated play area that is safe and enclosed. This can be a room or a section of your home where your rabbit can explore without encountering hazards.

Supervised Interaction: When allowing your rabbit to roam free, supervise them closely. Keep an eye on their behavior and ensure that they are not getting into anything unsafe or destructive.

Ultimately, the best approach may combine both cage and free-range living. A spacious cage for resting and safety, along with supervised free-range time, can provide your rabbit with a balanced environment.

Essential Supplies: Bedding, Hiding Spots, and Toys

Creating a rabbit-friendly living space involves providing the right supplies to keep your pet comfortable and entertained.

1. Bedding:

- Choose bedding that is safe and absorbent. Avoid cedar or pine shavings, as they can be toxic. Instead, opt for paper-based bedding, aspen shavings, or straw.
- Ensure that the bedding is deep enough to absorb moisture and provide warmth, while also allowing for easy cleaning.

Bedding Maintenance: Change bedding regularly to keep the living area clean and odor-free. Spot clean daily and do a thorough cleaning weekly to maintain hygiene.

- **Bedding Alternatives:** In addition to paper-based bedding, you can also consider using fleece blankets or towels, which can be washed regularly.

2. Hiding Spots:

- Rabbits are prey animals and require safe spaces to retreat when they feel threatened or stressed. Providing hiding spots can help them feel secure.
- Create hiding spots using cardboard boxes, tunnels, or commercially available rabbit hides. Ensure these areas are quiet and away from disturbances.

Creative Hiding Spots: Use items like cardboard boxes, tunnels made of cardboard or plastic, and even small pet tents to create diverse hiding spaces. You can also create a "bunny castle" with multiple levels for exploration.

Observation: Observe where your rabbit prefers to hide. This can give you insight into their personality and comfort level.

3. Toys:

- Keeping your rabbit mentally stimulated is crucial. Provide a variety of toys, such as chew toys, puzzle feeders, and safe wooden items to chew on.
- Rotate toys regularly to maintain your rabbit's interest and prevent boredom. Interactive toys that encourage foraging can also be beneficial.

DIY Toys: You can create homemade toys using safe materials. For example, cardboard tubes from paper towels or toilet paper can be filled with hay or treats for added excitement.

Interactive Play: Engage with your rabbit using toys that require them to think or work for their treats. Puzzle toys or treat mazes encourage physical and mental activity.

Safety Considerations

Ensuring your rabbit's safety in its environment is critical. Here are key safety measures to take when setting up your rabbit's home.

Rabbit-proofing your home and garden

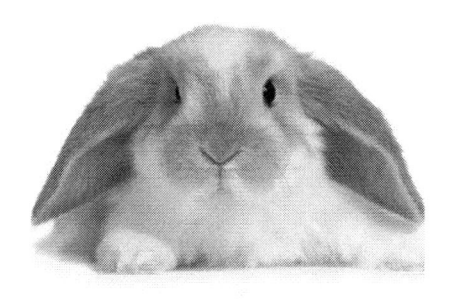

1. Furniture Protection:

- Consider using protective covers on furniture legs or edges to prevent chewing and damage. You can also use baby gates to block off areas that are off-limits.
- Move furniture and small items that could be knocked over or chewed on to prevent accidents. Keep items such as shoes, books, and clothes out of reach.

2. Cords and Cables:

- Rabbits love to chew, and exposed electrical cords can pose a serious hazard. Use cord protectors or hide cords behind furniture to minimize the risk of chewing.
- Use cord wraps or tubing designed to protect electrical cords. You can also secure cords along walls or behind furniture to keep them out of reach.

3. Outdoor Safety:

If your rabbit spends time outdoors, ensure that the area is secure. Enclose the garden with fencing that is tall enough to prevent jumping and deep enough to deter digging.

4. Toxic Plants:

Many common houseplants and garden plants are toxic to rabbits. Familiarize yourself with plants that are safe and those that are harmful. Research and create a comprehensive list of both safe and toxic plants. Many online resources and vet clinics provide databases of plants that are safe for rabbits.

Some common toxic plants include:

- Lilies

- Azaleas
- Poinsettias
- Ivy

If you have plants in your home or garden, consider removing or relocating toxic varieties.

5. Open Windows and Doors:

Ensure that windows and doors are secured to prevent your rabbit from escaping. Always supervise your rabbit when they are outside, as they can be quick to dart away.

Identifying Toxic Plants and Hazards

1. Research Safe Plants:

Create a list of safe plants for your home and garden. Safe options include:

- Basil
- Parsley
- Clover
- Timothy hay

Always double-check before introducing new plants to your environment.

2. Regular Inspections:

Periodically inspect your home and garden for potential hazards. Look for items that could be harmful, such as cleaning supplies, chemicals, or small choking hazards.

3. Chemical Safety:

Store cleaning supplies, pesticides, and other chemicals in locked cabinets or high shelves to prevent access. Always use rabbit-safe products for cleaning and gardening.

4. Regular Training:

Train your rabbit to understand boundaries. For instance, if there are areas or items you don't want them to access, gently redirect them when they approach those spots.

5. Educate Family Members:

Make sure everyone in your household understands the importance of rabbit safety. Teach family members the appropriate ways to interact with and handle your rabbit.

Additional Considerations for a Rabbit-Friendly Home

Temperature Control: Rabbits are sensitive to temperature extremes. Ensure that their living space is kept at a comfortable temperature, ideally between 60°F and 70°F. Avoid placing their cage in direct sunlight or near heating vents.

Social Interaction: Spend time daily interacting with your rabbit. Regular petting, gentle handling, and playtime are vital for building trust and a strong bond. Recognize their body language to understand when they want attention or when they prefer to be left alone.

Routine and Structure: Establishing a routine helps rabbits feel secure. Regular feeding times, play sessions, and clean-up schedules can create a predictable environment that reduces stress.

By carefully considering the layout of your rabbit's living space, providing essential supplies, and implementing safety measures, you can create an environment that promotes physical health, mental stimulation, and overall happiness for your rabbit. In doing so, you'll set the foundation for a long and fulfilling companionship.

Chapter Summary

In summary, setting up a rabbit-friendly home requires careful consideration of living arrangements, essential supplies, and safety measures. By providing a comfortable environment with proper bedding, hiding spots, and toys, along with implementing safety precautions, you can create a nurturing space where your rabbit can thrive. A well-prepared home will not only enhance your rabbit's quality of life but also strengthen the bond between you and your beloved pet.

CHAPTER 4
NUTRITION ESSENTIALS FOR YOUR RABBIT

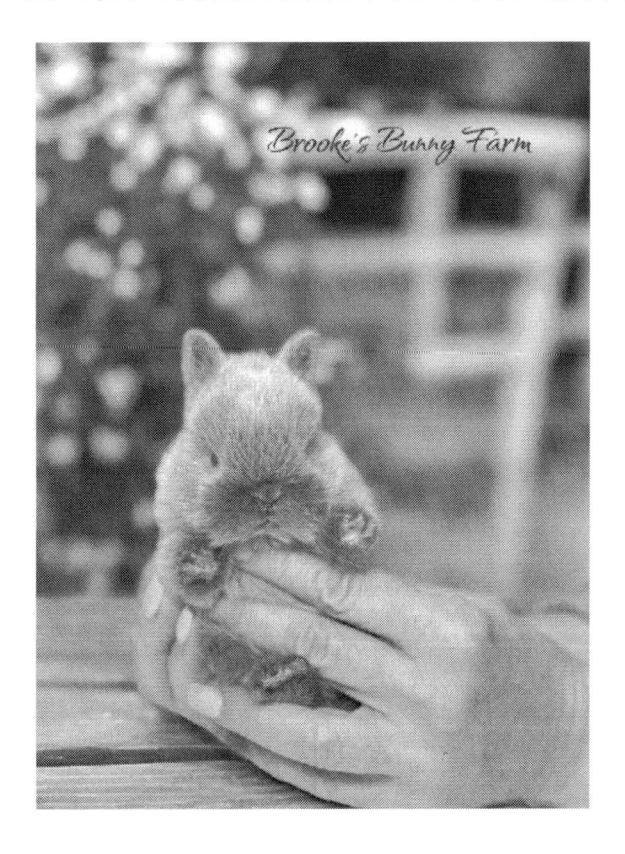

Providing your rabbit with a well-balanced diet is crucial for its health and longevity. Understanding the specific dietary needs of rabbits, including the importance of various food types and the role of supplements, will help you create a nutritious feeding plan. This chapter will cover the essential components of a rabbit's diet, safe and unsafe foods, and the use of supplements for optimal health.

Understanding a Rabbit's Dietary Needs

Rabbits are herbivores with unique dietary requirements that must be met to maintain their health. A balanced diet is essential for proper digestion, dental health, and overall well-being.

Importance of Hay, Fresh Vegetables, and Pellets

1. Hay:

Primary Food Source: Hay should constitute the majority of your rabbit's diet, ideally 80% or more. It provides essential fiber that aids in digestion and helps prevent gastrointestinal issues.

Types of Hay: The best options include:

Timothy Hay: The go-to choice for adult rabbits, it promotes dental health and provides the necessary fiber to aid digestion. High in fiber and low in protein, making it ideal for adult rabbits.

Orchard Grass Hay: A softer alternative that is also high in fiber.

Meadow Hay: Offers a mix of grasses and plants, providing variety and nutrients. It is often more palatable for picky eaters.

Feeding Tips: Ensure that hay is fresh, free from mold or dust, and available at all times. Your rabbit should have constant access to hay to encourage natural chewing behaviors.

Alfalfa Hay: High in protein and calcium, alfalfa hay is suitable for young rabbits, pregnant or nursing females, but should be limited for adult rabbits due to its richness.

Storage and Freshness: Store hay in a cool, dry place and keep it off the ground to prevent mold. Always check for freshness before feeding, as moldy hay can lead to respiratory issues.

2. Fresh Vegetables:

Daily Serving: Fresh vegetables should make up about 10-15% of your rabbit's diet. These provide essential vitamins and minerals. Aim for about 1 cup of fresh vegetables per 2 pounds of body weight. Always introduce vegetables gradually to avoid digestive upset.

Variety is Key: Rotate different types of vegetables to ensure a well-rounded intake of nutrients. This keeps meals interesting and encourages exploration of new tastes.

Limit Starchy Vegetables: Foods like corn, potatoes, and peas should be offered sparingly due to their higher starch content, which can lead to gastrointestinal problems.

Safe Vegetables: Some great options include:

- Leafy greens such as romaine lettuce, kale, and cilantro.
- Non-leafy vegetables like bell peppers, carrots (in moderation), and cucumber.

Introducing New Vegetables: Introduce new vegetables gradually to monitor for any digestive upset. Always wash vegetables thoroughly to remove pesticides and chemicals.

3. Pellets:

Supplementary Food: High-quality rabbit pellets can provide additional nutrients but should be fed in moderation (around 5-10% of the diet).

Choosing Pellets: Look for pellets that are high in fiber (at least 18%) and low in protein (around 16%) and calcium. Avoid pellets with added seeds, nuts, or dried fruits, as these can be high in fat and sugar and cause health issues.

Feeding Guidelines: Follow the feeding recommendations on the packaging based on your rabbit's weight and age. Overfeeding pellets can lead to obesity and related health issues.

Transitioning Pellets: If switching brands, do so gradually over a week to allow your rabbit's digestive system to adjust without causing stress or digestive upset.

Safe and Unsafe Foods for Rabbits

Understanding which foods are safe and which to avoid is crucial for your rabbit's health.

1. Safe Foods:

Fresh Vegetables: As mentioned earlier, leafy greens and certain non-leafy vegetables are safe. Offer a mix of greens daily. Some safe options include arugula, bok choy, and endive. These provide essential nutrients without excessive calories.

Fruits: Fruits should be given as occasional treats due to high sugar content. Safe options include apples (without seeds), blueberries, strawberries, and bananas. Limit fruits to about 1-2 tablespoons per

5 pounds of body weight. Remember to remove seeds and pits from fruits before offering them to your rabbit.

Certain Herbs: Parsley, basil, and dill are safe and can be offered as treats.

2. Unsafe Foods:

Toxic Plants: Familiarize yourself with common household plants that are toxic to rabbits, such as:

Pothos: Causes gastrointestinal distress.

Philodendron: Can lead to oral irritation and vomiting.

Human Food: Avoid any processed or sugary foods, as these can lead to obesity and other health issues. Foods like chocolate, caffeine, and alcohol are also toxic to rabbits.

Toxic Vegetables: Avoid feeding rabbits potatoes, onions, garlic, and rhubarb, as these can be harmful.

Certain Fruits: Cherries, grapes, and citrus fruits should be avoided due to their high sugar and acidity levels.

Processed Foods: Never feed your rabbit processed foods, bread, crackers, cookies, or any human food that is not specifically designed for rabbits.

Toxic Plants: Be aware of toxic plants, including lilies, azaleas, and poinsettias.

A comprehensive list of safe and unsafe foods should be kept handy for quick reference, ensuring your rabbit's diet remains safe and healthy. For quick results google search "Unsafe foods for Rabbits" and you'll find about 100 lists with pictures you can print and hang on your refrigerator.

Supplements for Optimal Health

While a balanced diet of hay, fresh vegetables, and pellets fulfills most of your rabbit's nutritional needs, certain conditions may necessitate the use of supplements.

Overview of Vitamins and Minerals

Rabbits require various vitamins and minerals for overall health:

1. Calcium: Essential for bone health but should be balanced with phosphorus. Excess calcium can lead to urinary problems.

2. Vitamin A: Important for vision and immune function. It is typically obtained from fresh greens.

3. B Vitamins: Necessary for energy metabolism and overall well-being. These can be found in hay and greens.

4. Fiber: While not a vitamin or mineral, fiber is crucial for digestive health. A high-fiber diet prevents issues like GI stasis.

When and How to Use Supplements

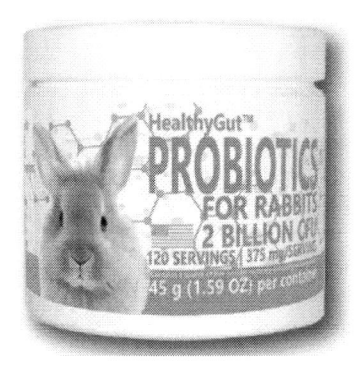

1. Determining Need:

Signs of Nutritional Deficiency: Look for signs like lethargy, poor coat condition, or changes in behavior that may indicate nutritional deficiencies. If you notice these signs, consult a veterinarian for guidance.

Routine Health Checks: Regular veterinary check-ups will help identify nutritional needs based on your rabbit's age, weight, and overall health status.

Consult a Veterinarian: Before introducing any supplements, consult with a veterinarian who specializes in rabbits. They can assess your rabbit's health and dietary needs.

Health Conditions: Certain health conditions, such as dental issues or gastrointestinal problems, may require specific supplements.

2. Types of Supplements:

Fiber Supplements: If your rabbit struggles with digestion, fiber supplements such as psyllium husk can help. However, this should be discussed with a veterinarian.

Herbal Supplements: Some herbal blends can support digestive health and overall wellness. Always consult with a vet before introducing herbal supplements to ensure they are safe and appropriate.

Vitamin Supplements: Commercially available vitamin supplements can help if your rabbit is not getting enough nutrients from its diet.

Probiotics: These can support digestive health, especially after antibiotic treatment or during digestive upset.

Calcium Supplements: If your rabbit is not getting enough calcium through its diet, a vet may recommend a calcium supplement, but this should be approached with caution to avoid excess.

3. Administration:

Consistency: Administer supplements consistently, either daily or as directed, to ensure your rabbit receives the intended benefits.

Monitoring Effects: After introducing a new supplement, monitor your rabbit's behavior and health closely. Look for improvements or any signs of adverse reactions.

Follow Dosage Instructions: Always adhere to the recommended dosage on the supplement packaging or as directed by your veterinarian.

Mixing with Food: Many supplements can be mixed with food to encourage your rabbit to consume them. Ensure that the supplement is palatable to your rabbit.

Additional Nutritional Considerations

Hydration: Fresh, clean water should always be available. Rabbits can be prone to dehydration, especially in warmer weather. Consider using a water bowl instead of a bottle, as some rabbits prefer drinking from a bowl.

Weight Management: Monitor your rabbit's weight regularly. Adjust their diet as needed based on their activity level, age, and health status. Obesity can lead to serious health issues, including arthritis and heart disease.

Feeding Routine: Establish a consistent feeding routine to help your rabbit feel secure and comfortable. Feed them at the same times each day to create a sense of stability.

Behavioral Feeding: Encourage foraging behaviors by hiding small amounts of hay or pellets around their living space. This stimulates their natural instincts and keeps them engaged.

Adjusting Diets for Age and Health: Young rabbits, adult rabbits, and seniors have different dietary needs. For instance, older rabbits may require softer foods and more frequent dental check-ups due to wear on their teeth.

Chapter Summary

In summary, understanding and meeting your rabbit's nutritional needs is essential for their health and happiness. A diet primarily composed of high-quality hay, complemented by fresh vegetables and limited pellets, will provide the necessary nutrients for your rabbit's well-being. Be mindful of safe and unsafe foods, and consider the use of supplements when necessary, always in consultation with a veterinarian. By fostering healthy eating habits and ensuring a balanced diet, you can significantly enhance your rabbit's quality of life and promote longevity.

CHAPTER 5
LITTER BOX TRAINING YOUR RABBIT

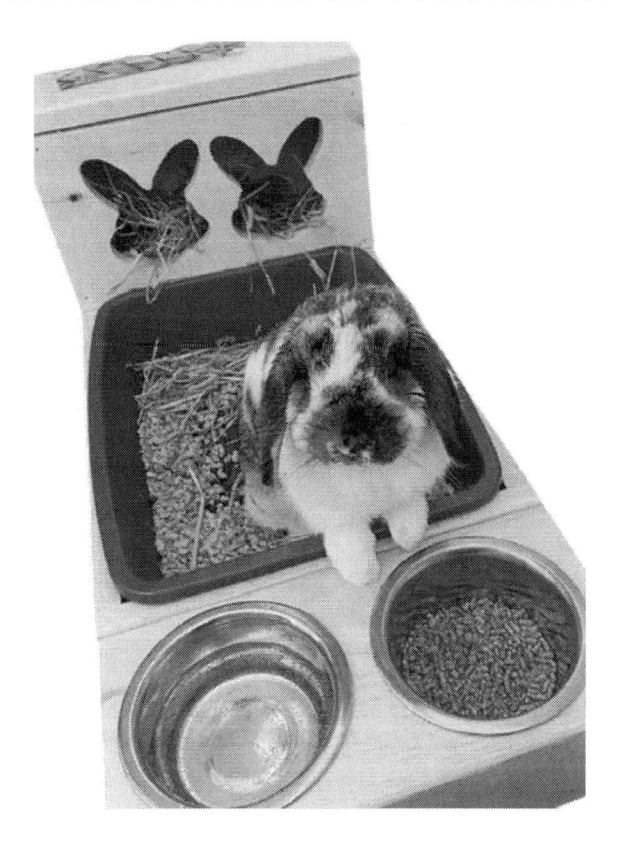

Litter box training is an essential aspect of rabbit care that contributes significantly to a clean and harmonious living environment. Unlike cats, rabbits require a bit more guidance when it comes to using a litter box, but with patience and the right approach, most rabbits can be successfully trained. This chapter will cover the basics of litter box training your rabbit, including how to choose the right litter and box size, the steps to train your rabbit, and common challenges you may face along with their solutions.

The Basics of Litter Box Training

Choosing the Right Litter & Box Size

1. Choosing the Right Litter:

Safe Materials: Select a litter that is safe for rabbits. Avoid clumping litters made from clay, as they can be harmful if ingested.

Instead, opt for:

Paper-based Litter: This type is absorbent, dust-free, and safe for rabbits. Brands like Carefresh or Yesterday's News are popular choices.

Hemp Litter: Made from hemp fibers, this option is biodegradable, absorbent, and has a pleasant odor.

Wood Pellets: Non-toxic wood pellets (like those made from aspen or pine) can also be used, though they should be kept dry since they can expand when wet.

Avoid Toxic Materials: Stay away from cedar and pine shavings, as the oils in these woods can be harmful to rabbits.

2. Choosing the Right Box Size:

Box Size: The litter box should be spacious enough for your rabbit to enter, turn around, and lie down comfortably. A good size for a small to medium rabbit is at least 24 inches long and 18 inches wide. Larger breeds may require a bigger box.

Design: Choose a box with low sides for easy entry, especially for younger or older rabbits. Some owners prefer covered litter boxes for odor control, but ensure your rabbit feels comfortable and safe inside.

Accessibility: Place the litter box in an area where your rabbit spends most of its time. This can be near its cage or in a favorite corner of the room.

Steps to Successfully Train Your Rabbit

1. Establish a Routine:

Rabbits thrive on routine. Offer meals at the same time each day and allow your rabbit to use the litter box following meals. This is often when they feel the need to eliminate.

2. Introduce the Litter Box:

- Place your rabbit inside the litter box gently. Allow them to explore it, and do not force them to stay in.
- Use a small amount of litter to line the bottom of the box. You can also add some of your rabbit's droppings to the box to encourage them to recognize the box as the proper place to eliminate.

3. Encourage Use:

- After meals and when you notice signs that your rabbit needs to go (such as circling or sniffing), place them in the litter box.
- Reward your rabbit with gentle praise or a small treat immediately after they use the box successfully. Positive reinforcement helps them associate the box with good experiences.

4. Be Patient and Consistent:

Training may take time, and accidents are normal. Stay patient and consistent in your training efforts. If your rabbit eliminates outside the box, gently pick them up and place them back in the box without scolding.

5. Clean Up Accidents Properly:

Clean any areas where your rabbit has eliminated outside of the box with an enzyme cleaner to remove odors. This helps prevent your rabbit from returning to the same spot to eliminate again.

6. Monitor Progress:

Keep track of your rabbit's progress. Most rabbits will become proficient in litter box use within a few weeks, while some may take longer. Adjust your training approach as needed based on your rabbit's behavior.

Common Challenges and Solutions

Despite your best efforts, you may encounter challenges during the litter box training process. Here are some common issues and their solutions:

Troubleshooting Accidents

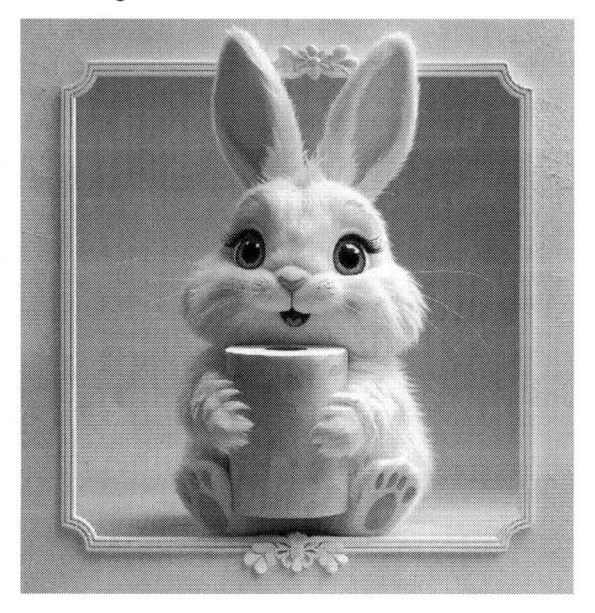

1. Accidents Outside the Box:

Possible Causes: Accidents can occur for several reasons, including stress, illness, or an unclean box.

Solution: Ensure the litter box is clean and filled with fresh litter. If accidents persist, consider whether your rabbit is experiencing stress from changes in the environment or routine. Address any stressors to help your rabbit feel secure.

2. Inconsistent Use:

Possible Causes: If your rabbit is not consistently using the litter box, it could be due to an improperly sized box, an unsuitable location, or the type of litter used.

Solution: Evaluate the size and location of the box. Experiment with different litter types to see which one your rabbit prefers. Some rabbits may also prefer having multiple litter boxes if they have a large living space.

3. Marking Territory:

Possible Causes: Rabbits may mark their territory by urinating or leaving droppings in various areas. This behavior is more common in unspayed or unneutered rabbits.

Solution: Consider spaying or neutering your rabbit, which often reduces territorial marking behavior. Additionally, provide plenty of opportunities for your rabbit to explore and feel secure in their space.

Behavioral Issues

1. Refusing to Use the Litter Box:

Possible Causes: If your rabbit is refusing to use the litter box, it may be due to discomfort with the box, the litter, or health issues.

Solution: Reassess the litter box setup. Ensure it's clean, adequately sized, and in a quiet area. If your rabbit continues to refuse the box, consult a veterinarian to rule out potential health problems, such as urinary tract infections.

2. Litter Box Grazing:

Possible Causes: Some rabbits may enjoy munching on the litter, especially if it contains hay or is made of edible materials.

Solution: Monitor your rabbit's behavior and consider switching to a non-edible litter type if they are consuming too much litter. Ensure they have access to plenty of hay and fresh vegetables to satisfy their chewing instincts.

3. Stress and Anxiety:

Possible Causes: Changes in the environment, loud noises, or other household pets can cause stress for your rabbit, leading to litter box issues.

Solution: Create a safe and quiet space for your rabbit. Consider providing hiding spots and vertical spaces to help them feel secure. Spend time interacting with your rabbit to build trust and reduce anxiety.

Additional Tips for Successful Litter Box Training

1. Understanding Rabbit Behavior:

Natural Instincts: Rabbits prefer to eliminate in specific areas. By recognizing this behavior, you can strategically place litter boxes in the spots where your rabbit tends to go. If you notice them consistently using a corner of the room, consider placing the litter box there.

Observation: Spend time observing your rabbit's habits. This will help you understand their elimination patterns and reinforce the training process.

2. Using Multiple Litter Boxes:

For Larger Spaces: If your rabbit has access to a large area or multiple rooms, consider placing multiple litter boxes. This reduces the likelihood of accidents and gives your rabbit convenient options for elimination.

Traveling with Your Rabbit: If you take your rabbit on trips or to different locations, bring a portable litter box to help them maintain their routine.

3. Creating a Positive Association:

Desensitization: If your rabbit seems hesitant to use the litter box, gently encourage them by placing treats or favorite toys inside the box. This can help create a positive association and encourage exploration.

Calming Aids: If your rabbit is particularly anxious, consider using calming aids such as herbal supplements or pheromone sprays designed for rabbits to create a soothing environment.

Detailed Examination of Behavioral Issues

1. Understanding Accidental Elimination:

Young Rabbits: Young rabbits may have less control over their bladder and bowels, leading to more accidents. Patience is vital during this phase. Gradually, as they grow and mature, they will likely become more reliable in using the litter box.

Senior Rabbits: Older rabbits may face health issues such as arthritis, which can make it difficult for them to access their litter box. In this case, consider using a box with lower sides or placing multiple boxes closer to their resting areas.

2. Addressing Territorial Marking:

Spaying/Neutering: This is one of the most effective ways to reduce territorial marking behavior. If your rabbit has not been spayed or neutered, consult your veterinarian about the benefits of the procedure.

Environmental Enrichment: Providing plenty of toys, tunnels, and areas to explore can help reduce territorial tendencies and make your rabbit feel more secure in their environment.

3. Identifying Stressors:

Changes in Routine: Any significant changes in your household, such as moving, new pets, or new family members, can stress your rabbit. Try to maintain a consistent routine and gradually introduce changes to help them adjust.

Noise Sensitivity: Some rabbits are sensitive to loud noises. If your rabbit is reacting to household sounds (like vacuuming or construction noise), try to create a quiet, safe space where they can retreat during these times.

Maintaining a Healthy Litter Box Environment

1. Regular Cleaning:

Daily Maintenance: Clean the litter box daily by removing soiled litter and droppings. This prevents odors and keeps the box inviting for your rabbit.

Deep Cleaning: Every week, fully empty the litter box, wash it with a mild, rabbit-safe detergent, and rinse thoroughly. This helps eliminate any lingering odors and bacteria.

2. Choosing the Right Location:

Quiet and Safe Spot: The litter box should be placed in a quiet area away from high-traffic zones or loud appliances. Rabbits prefer privacy when they eliminate.

Avoiding Food Areas: Position the litter box away from your rabbit's food and water bowls. Rabbits generally do not like to eliminate near their eating areas.

3. Monitoring Litter Usage:

Health Indicators: Keep an eye on your rabbit's litter box habits. Changes in their elimination patterns, such as increased frequency or a sudden decrease, can indicate health issues. **(If you notice anything unusual, consult your veterinarian).**

Tracking Progress: Document your rabbit's litter box usage to identify any patterns over time. This can help you fine-tune your training approach and address any ongoing issues.

Encouraging Positive Behavior

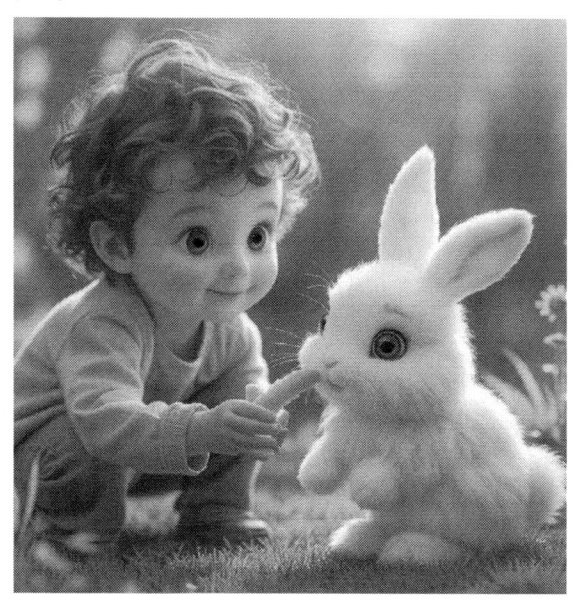

1. Reward System:

Use Treats: Every time your rabbit uses the litter box successfully, reward them with a small treat or extra attention. This reinforces the behavior positively.

Verbal Praise: Use a gentle, encouraging tone when your rabbit uses the litter box. Consistent praise helps them associate the action with positive reinforcement.

2. Patience and Consistency:

Training Takes Time: Remember that litter box training is a process. Some rabbits may grasp it quickly, while others may take longer. Consistency in your approach and patience in your training efforts are key.

Avoid Punishment: Never scold or punish your rabbit for accidents. This can create fear and anxiety, making them less likely to use the litter box. Instead, focus on positive reinforcement.

Chapter Summary

Litter box training your rabbit is a rewarding journey that requires understanding, patience, and consistency. By choosing the right litter, providing an appropriately sized box, and following structured training steps, you can teach your rabbit to use the litter box effectively. Understanding and addressing common challenges, maintaining a clean litter box environment, and encouraging positive behaviors will help create a successful training experience.

With dedication, you can foster a clean living space for both you and your rabbit while strengthening the bond between you. A well-trained rabbit not only contributes to a tidier home but also leads to a happier, healthier life for your furry friend.

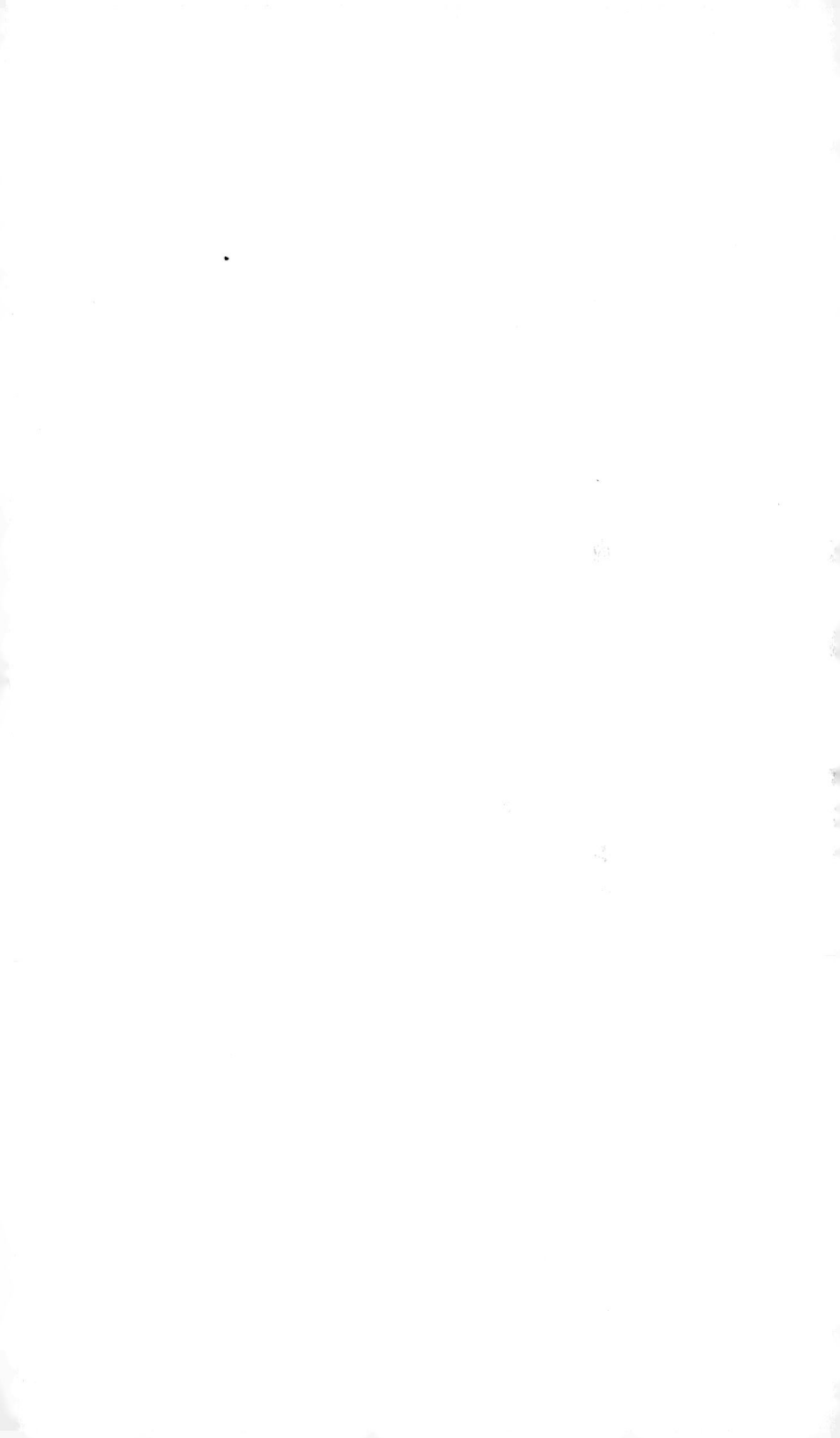

CHAPTER 6
HEALTH AND WELLNESS

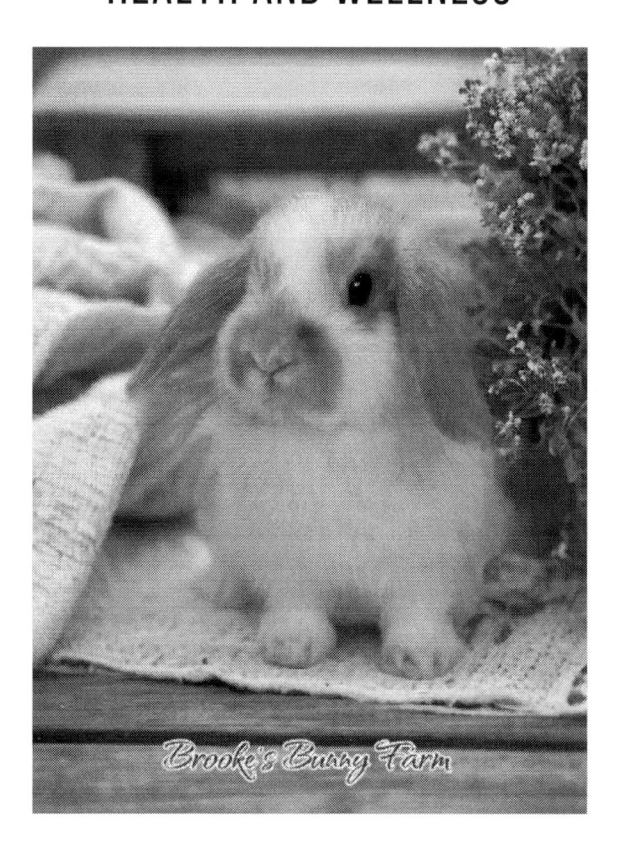

Maintaining your rabbit's health and wellness is crucial for ensuring a long, happy life. This chapter will cover the importance of routine veterinary care, including spaying/neutering and vaccinations, how to recognize signs of illness in rabbits, and preventative health measures like grooming, dental care, and maintaining a healthy weight.

Routine Veterinary Care

Importance of Spaying/Neutering and Vaccinations

1. Spaying/Neutering:

What is Spaying/Neutering? Spaying refers to the surgical removal of a female rabbit's reproductive organs, while neutering refers to the removal of a male rabbit's testicles. This procedure is commonly performed by a veterinarian.

Health Benefits:

Reduced Cancer Risk: Spaying female rabbits significantly reduces the risk of uterine cancer, which is common in unspayed females. Neutering male rabbits can prevent testicular cancer and reduce the risk of prostate issues.

Behavioral Improvements: Spayed and neutered rabbits are often calmer and less aggressive. They are less likely to exhibit territorial behaviors, such as spraying or marking their territory with urine. In addition to reducing aggression and territorial marking, spaying and neutering can improve your rabbit's overall demeanor. Spayed females are less likely to exhibit nesting behavior, which can be stressful for both the rabbit and the owner. Neutered males tend to be more affectionate and social.

Reduced Overpopulation: Spaying and neutering help control the rabbit population, preventing unwanted litters and contributing to fewer rabbits in shelters.

When to Spay/Neuter: Ideally, rabbits should be spayed or neutered between 4 to 6 months of age. However, consult your veterinarian for personalized recommendations based on your rabbit's health and breed.

Post-Surgical Care: After the procedure, monitor your rabbit for any signs of discomfort, such as lethargy or refusal to eat. Provide a quiet, cushioned space for recovery, and follow your veterinarian's instructions for aftercare, which may include pain management and dietary adjustments.

Timing of Surgery: Discuss with your veterinarian the best time for spaying or neutering. While the typical age is around 4-6 months, some veterinarians may recommend doing it earlier or later based on your rabbit's health and breed.

2. Vaccinations:

Essential Vaccines: Vaccinations are critical for protecting rabbits from serious diseases. Common vaccinations include:

Myxomatosis: A viral disease that is often fatal; vaccination is essential, especially in areas where the disease is prevalent.

Rabbit Hemorrhagic Disease (RHD): This highly contagious and fatal virus can spread quickly among rabbits. Vaccination is crucial, particularly if your rabbit is at risk of exposure.

Consulting Your Veterinarian: Discuss your rabbit's vaccination schedule with your veterinarian. They will recommend the appropriate vaccines based on your rabbit's age, health, and lifestyle.

Types of Vaccines: In some regions, additional vaccines may be recommended based on local disease prevalence. For example, in areas where RHDV2 is a concern, specific vaccines targeting this strain may be advised.

Vaccination Schedule: Keep a record of your rabbit's vaccinations and schedule regular check-ups. Many vaccines require boosters, so staying on top of these appointments is essential for your rabbit's health.

Recognizing signs of illness in rabbits

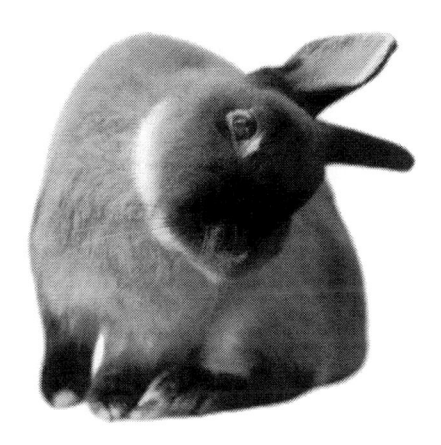

Being aware of the signs of illness in rabbits is essential for early detection and treatment. Rabbits are prey animals and may hide their symptoms until a condition becomes severe. Here are some key signs to watch for:

1. Changes in Appetite:

A sudden decrease or complete loss of appetite can indicate dental problems, gastrointestinal stasis, or illness. If your rabbit is not eating, consult a veterinarian immediately.

Gastrointestinal Stasis: A common issue in rabbits is gastrointestinal stasis, characterized by a decrease in appetite and changes in droppings. This condition can be life-threatening if not addressed promptly. If your rabbit stops eating or shows a significant reduction in food intake, contact your veterinarian immediately.

2. Altered Behavior:

Lethargy, unusual aggression, or withdrawal from interactions can signal illness or discomfort. Changes in grooming habits, such as unkempt fur, can also indicate health issues.

Social Withdrawal: If your rabbit suddenly becomes less social or interactive, it may be a sign of distress or illness. Monitor for other symptoms, such as changes in eating habits or litter box usage.

Pain Indicators: Rabbits often hide pain well. Signs of pain can include grinding teeth, a hunched posture, or a reluctance to move. If you notice these behaviors, seek veterinary assistance.

3. Changes in Droppings:

Monitor your rabbit's droppings regularly. Small, hard, or absent fecal pellets can indicate gastrointestinal issues. Soft, watery droppings may suggest a digestive upset or parasitic infection.

Normal vs. Abnormal Droppings: Healthy rabbit droppings should be round, firm, and dark brown. Any significant changes in size, shape, or consistency should prompt a veterinary visit. For example, small, hard pellets may indicate dehydration or a lack of fiber, while soft or watery droppings can signify digestive upset.

Monitoring Urination: Changes in urination, such as increased frequency or straining, can indicate a urinary tract infection or bladder stones. Keep an eye on your rabbit's litter box for changes.

Diarrhea: Diarrhea can result from dietary changes, eating spoiled food, or infections. It can lead to dehydration and requires prompt veterinary care.

4. Respiratory Symptoms:

Watch for signs of respiratory distress, including sneezing, nasal discharge, or labored breathing. These symptoms can indicate infections or other respiratory conditions that require veterinary attention.

Signs of Infection: If your rabbit exhibits nasal discharge, coughing, or wheezing, it may indicate a respiratory infection, such as Pasteurella. Early veterinary intervention is crucial to prevent complications.

5. Dental Issues:

Signs of dental problems can include drooling, difficulty eating, or pawing at the mouth. Overgrown teeth can lead to serious complications and should be addressed promptly.

Malocclusion: This condition occurs when the teeth don't align properly, causing them to rub against the gums and other teeth, resulting in pain and potential abscesses.

Preventing Dental Problems: To help prevent dental issues, provide plenty of chew toys and a diet high in fiber. Regularly check your rabbit's teeth for any signs of overgrowth or misalignment.

Veterinary Dental Care: If you suspect dental problems, your veterinarian can perform dental examinations and recommend treatments, which may include filing down overgrown teeth or addressing underlying issues.

6. Abnormal Posture or Movement:

If your rabbit is hunching, showing signs of pain, or limping, it may be experiencing discomfort or injury. Any abnormal posture should be evaluated by a veterinarian.

Signs of Injury: If your rabbit shows signs of limping or favoring a limb, it may have an injury. Observe their movements closely and consult a veterinarian if you notice any irregularities.

7. Ear Problems:

Ear Mites: These parasites can cause itching, inflammation, and discomfort in the ears. Symptoms include excessive scratching and head shaking.

Ear Infections: Infections can result from bacterial or fungal pathogens, leading to pain and potential hearing loss.

8. Skin Problems:

Fleas and Ticks: External parasites can cause skin irritation and lead to more serious infections if not treated.

Dermatitis: Skin irritation can occur due to allergies, poor hygiene, or infections, leading to redness, itching, and hair loss.

9. Heatstroke:

Rabbits are sensitive to heat and can suffer from heatstroke if exposed to high temperatures without adequate ventilation or shade. Symptoms include panting, lethargy, and a rapid heartbeat.

10. Reproductive Health Issues:

Unspayed female rabbits are at risk of developing uterine cancer and other reproductive system problems. Spaying and neutering are recommended to prevent such issues and reduce unwanted litters.

Preventative Health Measures:

Grooming

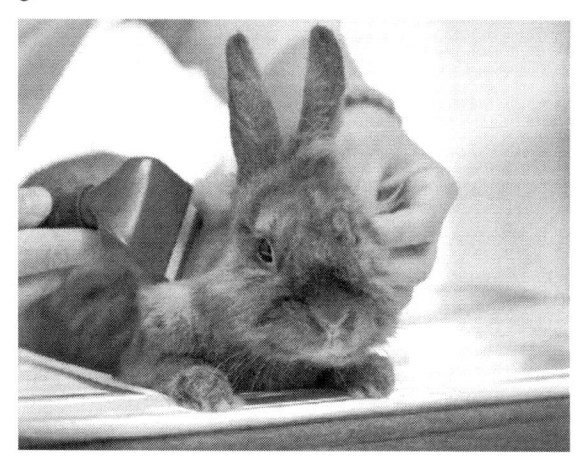

1. Importance of Grooming:

Regular grooming is essential for maintaining your rabbit's coat and skin health. It helps remove loose fur, dirt, and debris while also allowing you to check for any skin issues or parasites.

Grooming can reduce the risk of hairballs, especially in long-haired breeds, and helps prevent matting.

Seasonal Considerations: During shedding seasons (spring and fall), rabbits may require more frequent grooming to help remove excess fur and reduce the risk of hairballs. Monitor your rabbit's coat closely during these times.

Long-Haired vs. Short-Haired Rabbits: Long-haired breeds, such as Angoras, require daily grooming to prevent mats and tangles, while short-haired breeds may only need weekly brushing.

Importance of Nail Care: Regular nail trimming is essential for preventing overgrown nails, which can lead to discomfort and mobility issues. Overgrown nails can also curl and cause injury.

Trimming Techniques: Use specially designed rabbit nail clippers or human nail clippers. Trim only the tip of the nail to avoid cutting into the quick (the sensitive part containing blood vessels). If you're unsure, seek guidance from your veterinarian or a professional groomer.

2. Grooming Techniques:

Brush Regularly: Use a soft-bristled brush or a grooming glove to brush your rabbit's fur. Long-haired rabbits may require daily brushing, while short-haired rabbits can be groomed weekly.

Check Ears and Eyes: While grooming, examine your rabbit's ears for dirt or wax buildup and check their eyes for discharge or redness. Clean them gently with a damp cloth if needed.

Bathing: Rabbits generally do not require baths, as they groom themselves. If your rabbit gets dirty, it's best to spot clean with a damp cloth rather than giving a full bath.

Dental Care

1. Understanding Rabbit Dental Health:

Rabbits have continuously growing teeth, and proper dental care is essential to prevent overgrowth, malocclusion, and related health issues.

Dental problems can lead to pain, difficulty eating, and serious health complications.

2. Promoting Healthy Teeth:

Diet: Provide a diet rich in hay, which promotes natural chewing and helps wear down teeth. Avoid high-sugar or low-fiber foods that can contribute to dental issues.

Chew Toys: Offer safe chew toys made from untreated wood or hay-based products to encourage healthy chewing habits.

Checking for Overgrowth: Regularly check your rabbit's teeth for signs of overgrowth, such as uneven wear or sharp points. If your rabbit is reluctant to eat or shows signs of pain while chewing, consult a veterinarian.

Preventive Dental Care: Provide various chew toys to promote natural wear on teeth. Materials like untreated wood, hay cubes, and cardboard can be beneficial.

Regular Check-ups: Schedule regular veterinary check-ups to monitor your rabbit's dental health. Your veterinarian can perform dental examinations and file down overgrown teeth if necessary.

Maintaining a Healthy Weight

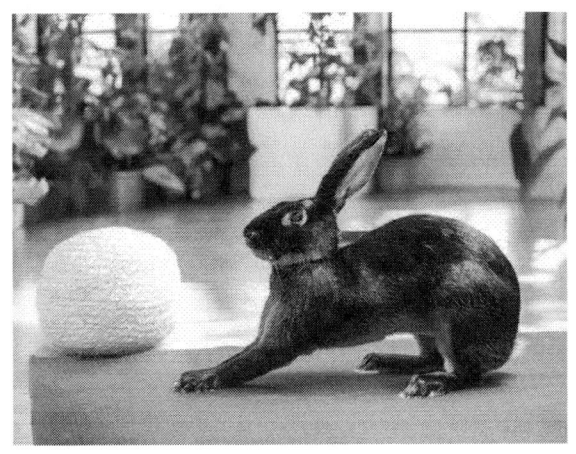

1. Understanding Ideal Weight:

Maintaining a healthy weight is crucial for your rabbit's overall health. Obesity can lead to serious health issues, including heart disease, arthritis, and gastrointestinal stasis.

Each rabbit breed has a different ideal weight range. Consult your veterinarian to determine the ideal weight for your specific breed.

Assessing Your Rabbit's Weight: Learn how to assess your rabbit's body condition by gently feeling their ribs and spine. You should be able to feel the ribs without excessive pressure, and there should be a slight waist when viewed from above.

Weight Management Plans: If your rabbit is overweight, work with your veterinarian to create a weight management plan that includes a balanced diet and increased exercise.

2. Monitoring Weight:

Weigh your rabbit regularly, ideally every month. Keep a log of their weight to track any changes over time.

If you notice significant weight gain or loss, consult your veterinarian to identify any underlying health issues.

Promoting Exercise:
Safe Play Areas: Create safe, enclosed spaces for your rabbit to explore and play. Use tunnels, ramps, and toys to encourage physical activity.

Interactive Play: Engage in interactive play with your rabbit using toys that stimulate their natural instincts, such as foraging toys or puzzle feeders.

3. Encouraging Healthy Habits:

Balanced Diet: Ensure your rabbit's diet is primarily composed of high-quality hay, fresh vegetables, and limited pellets. Avoid overfeeding and monitor treat intake.

Exercise: Provide ample opportunities for exercise and mental stimulation. Create a safe, enclosed space where your rabbit can roam and play. Encouraging natural behaviors, such as hopping and exploring, helps maintain a healthy weight.

Healthy Treat Options: Offer healthy treats in moderation. Small amounts of fresh fruits or vegetables can be rewarding, but avoid high-calorie treats like commercial rabbit snacks or sugary fruits.

Establishing Guidelines: Limit treats to no more than 10% of your rabbit's daily food intake to maintain a balanced diet.

4. Recognizing Obesity:

Signs of obesity in rabbits include difficulty grooming, a lack of mobility, and a noticeable layer of fat covering the ribs. Consult your veterinarian for guidance on creating a weight loss plan if needed.

Chapter Summary

Routine veterinary care and preventative health measures are vital for ensuring your rabbit's long-term health and wellness. Spaying or neutering and keeping up with vaccinations can prevent serious health issues, while recognizing signs of illness allows for early intervention. Regular grooming, dental care, and maintaining a healthy weight contribute to your rabbit's overall well-being.

By prioritizing your rabbit's health and wellness, you not only enhance their quality of life but also strengthen the bond between you and your furry companion. With proper care, your rabbit can enjoy a happy, healthy, and fulfilling life for many years to come.

Additionally, regular grooming, dental care, and maintaining a healthy weight contribute significantly to your rabbit's quality of life. By being proactive in your rabbit's health management, you can help ensure they lead a long, happy, and healthy life. Your commitment to their health not only enhances their well-being but also strengthens the bond between you and your furry companion, creating a fulfilling partnership for years to come.

CHAPTER 7
UNDERSTANDING RABBIT BEHAVIOR AND TRAINING TECHNIQUES

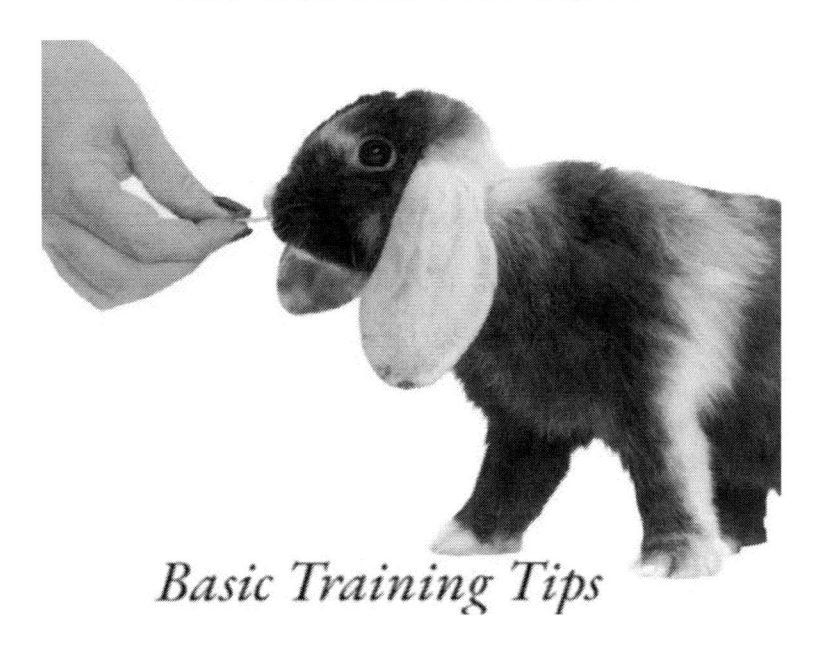

Basic Training Tips

Rabbits are intelligent and social animals that can learn a variety of commands and tricks, making them wonderful companions. Understanding rabbit behavior is key to successful training and fostering a positive relationship between you and your pet. This chapter will cover basic commands and tricks you can teach your rabbit and address common behavioral issues along with effective solutions.

Basic Commands and Tricks

Teaching Your Rabbit to Come, Stay, and Other Simple Commands

1. Understanding Your Rabbit's Learning Style:

Rabbits learn best through positive reinforcement, which means rewarding them for desired behaviors. This can include treats, verbal praise, or gentle petting. The key is to create a positive association with the behavior you want to encourage.

Consistency is crucial. Use the same cues and commands each time to help your rabbit learn effectively.

2. Teaching the "Come" Command:

Step 1: Choose a Quiet Space: Start in a quiet, distraction-free area where your rabbit feels comfortable.

Step 2: Use a Cue Word: Select a cue word like "come" or "here." Say the word clearly and in a friendly tone.

Step 3: Encourage Movement: While saying the cue, gently coax your rabbit towards you with a treat. You can also use their favorite toy to encourage movement.

Step 4: Reward: As soon as your rabbit approaches you, reward them immediately with a treat and praise them enthusiastically. This positive reinforcement will help them associate the cue with coming towards you.

Step 5: Practice: Repeat this process multiple times in short training sessions, gradually increasing the distance from which you call them. Consistency and patience are key.

3. Teaching the "Stay" Command:

Step 1: Get Your Rabbit's Attention: Start by having your rabbit in a sitting position close to you.

Step 2: Introduce the Command: Say "stay" in a calm and firm voice.

Step 3: Use a Hand Signal: Pair the verbal command with a hand signal, such as holding your hand out with your palm facing them.

Step 4: Move Away: Take a small step back while maintaining eye contact. If your rabbit stays in place, reward them immediately with a treat and praise.

Step 5: Gradually Increase Distance: As your rabbit becomes more comfortable with the command, gradually increase the distance and duration before rewarding. If they move, gently guide them back to the starting position and try again.

4. Teaching Other Simple Tricks:

"Hop Up": Encourage your rabbit to jump onto a surface, such as a low table or a designated spot. Use a treat to guide them and reward them when they successfully jump up.

"Spin": Hold a treat in front of your rabbit's nose and move it in a circle. As they follow the treat, say "spin" and reward them when they complete the turn.

"High Five": Encourage your rabbit to raise their paw by tapping it gently and offering a treat when they lift it. Use the command "high five" consistently to associate the action with the command.

5. Tips for Successful Training:

Short Sessions: Keep training sessions brief (5-10 minutes) to maintain your rabbit's attention and enthusiasm. Multiple short sessions throughout the day can be more effective than one long session.

Patience is Key: Every rabbit learns at their own pace. Be patient and avoid showing frustration. If your rabbit isn't catching on, take a break and try again later.

Use High-Value Treats: Use your rabbit's favorite treats as rewards to motivate them during training. Fresh vegetables or small pieces of fruit can work well, but keep treats small to avoid overfeeding.

Addressing Behavioral Issues

Solutions for Common Problems like Chewing and Digging

1. Understanding Chewing Behavior:

Natural Instinct: Chewing is a natural behavior for rabbits, as their teeth grow continuously. They chew to keep their teeth trimmed and to explore their environment.

Identifying Chewing Targets: Common targets include furniture, electrical cords, and houseplants. Identifying what your rabbit is chewing can help you redirect their behavior.

2. Solutions for Chewing:

Provide Chew Toys: Offer a variety of safe chew toys made from natural materials like untreated wood, hay-based toys, or cardboard. This provides an outlet for their chewing instinct.

Rabbit-Proof Your Home: Take measures to protect furniture and cords by using cord protectors, moving items out of reach, and providing designated areas where chewing is acceptable.

Redirect Behavior: If you catch your rabbit chewing on something inappropriate, redirect them to a chew toy or a designated chew area. Reward them when they choose the appropriate item.

3. Understanding Digging Behavior:

Instinctual Behavior: Digging is a natural behavior for rabbits that stems from their instincts to create burrows and find hiding spots. This behavior can also be a sign of boredom or excess energy.

Identifying Triggers: Observe when your rabbit digs—are they trying to get your attention, bored, or reacting to stress? Understanding the motivation can help address the behavior effectively.

4. Solutions for Digging:

Provide Digging Alternatives: Create a designated digging area using a shallow box filled with safe materials like shredded paper, hay, or soil. Encourage your rabbit to dig in this area by placing treats or toys inside.

Increase Exercise and Enrichment: Ensure your rabbit has plenty of opportunities for exercise and mental stimulation. Provide tunnels, climbing structures, and toys to keep them engaged and occupied.

Limit Stressors: If your rabbit digs when feeling anxious, ensure they have a safe and secure environment. Provide hiding spots and quiet areas where they can retreat when feeling stressed.

5. Addressing Other Common Behavioral Issues:

Nipping or Biting: If your rabbit nips at you, it may be a sign of playfulness or a desire for attention. Redirect this behavior by offering toys or treats instead of allowing them to nip. If biting is aggressive, consult a veterinarian or animal behaviorist.

Litter Box Issues: If your rabbit is not using the litter box consistently, evaluate the litter box setup and cleanliness. Ensure the box is large enough, filled with appropriate litter, and placed in a quiet area. Reinforce litter box use with positive reinforcement when they use it correctly.

Let's delve deeper into rabbit behavior, expanding on training techniques, providing more insights on addressing behavioral issues, and exploring additional aspects of rabbit care that relate to their behavior.

Advanced Training Techniques

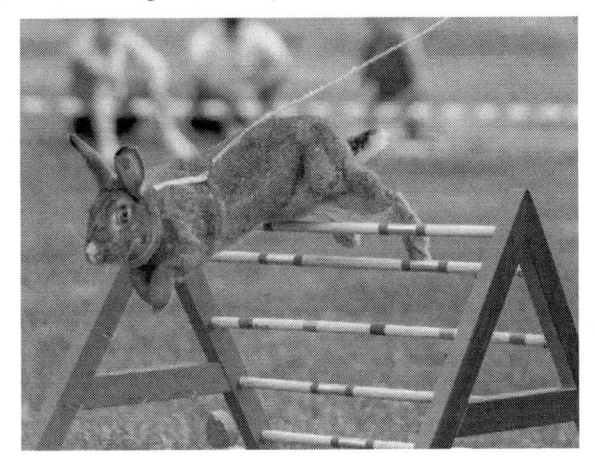

1. Clicker Training:

What is Clicker Training? Clicker training is a method of positive reinforcement that uses a sound (the click) to signal to the rabbit that they have performed the desired behavior correctly. This method can be highly effective for training rabbits.

Step-by-Step Guide:

Introduce the Clicker: Start by clicking the clicker and immediately giving your rabbit a treat. Repeat this several times so your rabbit associates the sound of the click with receiving a reward.

Add Commands: Once your rabbit understands that the click means a treat, you can begin to add commands. For example, when teaching "come," click and treat when your rabbit approaches you.

Create a Training Session: Use the clicker consistently during training sessions to reinforce desired behaviors. Remember to keep sessions short and fun.

2. Target Training:

What is Target Training? Target training involves teaching your rabbit to touch a specific object (the target) with their nose or paw. This can be useful for guiding your rabbit during training.

How to Implement Target Training:

Choose a Target: Use a small object, such as a wooden stick or a small ball.

Encourage Touching the Target: Hold the target close to your rabbit's nose. When they sniff or touch it, click the clicker (if using one) and reward them.

Increase Distance: Gradually increase the distance between the target and your rabbit, reinforcing the behavior as they follow the target.

3. Advanced Tricks:

"Jump Through a Hoop": Use a small hoop to train your rabbit to jump through. Start by placing the hoop on the ground and rewarding your rabbit for approaching it. Gradually lift the hoop as they become more confident.

"Weave Between Legs": Teach your rabbit to weave through your legs as you walk. Use treats to guide them and reward them for successfully navigating the course.

Dealing with Fearful or Timid Rabbits

1. Understanding Fearful Behavior:

Some rabbits may be naturally timid or have had negative experiences that make them fearful. Recognizing signs of fear—such as freezing, thumping, or hiding—can help you address their needs effectively.

2. Building Trust:

Create a Safe Space: Ensure your rabbit has a quiet, comfortable area where they can retreat when feeling anxious. This could be a cozy hideaway or a designated pen.

Gentle Interactions: Approach your rabbit calmly and gently. Avoid sudden movements or loud noises that may startle them. Allow your rabbit to come to you at their own pace.

Positive Reinforcement: Use treats and gentle praise to reward your rabbit for showing curiosity or bravery. This can help them associate positive experiences with new situations or interactions.

3. Gradual Exposure:

Slowly introduce your rabbit to new environments, people, or situations. Take baby steps and monitor their reactions. If they seem overwhelmed, back off and try again later.

Use treats to encourage exploration. Scatter treats in new areas to motivate your rabbit to investigate.

Socialization and Bonding

1. Importance of Socialization:

Socialization is crucial for helping your rabbit feel comfortable around people and other pets. A well-socialized rabbit is more likely to be calm and confident in various situations.

2. Interacting with Your Rabbit:

Daily Interaction: Spend time each day interacting with your rabbit. This can include gentle petting, talking, or simply sitting near them to build comfort.

Playtime: Engage in playtime that encourages interaction. Use toys, tunnels, and foraging games to stimulate your rabbit's mind and encourage bonding.

3. Introducing New Friends:

If you are considering adding another rabbit to your household, introduce them gradually and carefully. Ensure that both rabbits are spayed/neutered to prevent territorial behavior.

Use a neutral space for introductions, allowing the rabbits to interact without feeling threatened by established territory. Monitor their behavior and provide plenty of positive reinforcement for calm interactions.

Addressing Specific Behavioral Issues

1. Excessive Thumping:

Thumping is a natural behavior that rabbits use to signal alarm or discomfort. If your rabbit is thumping excessively, it may be a sign of stress or fear.

Solution: Identify potential stressors in their environment, such as loud noises or unfamiliar pets. Create a calm space where your rabbit can feel safe. Engage in gentle play or reward them for calm behavior to help reduce anxiety.

2. Boredom-Related Behaviors:

Rabbits can become bored if they lack mental stimulation, leading to destructive behaviors like digging or chewing.

Solution: Provide a variety of toys, tunnels, and interactive games to keep your rabbit engaged. Rotate toys regularly to maintain their interest. Foraging activities, where treats are hidden in hay or boxes, can also provide mental stimulation.

3. Inappropriate Elimination:

If your rabbit is not using the litter box consistently, it can be frustrating. Assess the litter box setup, cleanliness, and location.

Solution: Ensure the litter box is large enough, easily accessible, and filled with suitable litter. If accidents occur, clean the area thoroughly to remove odors. Reinforce proper litter box use with praise and treats when they use it correctly.

Chapter Summary

Understanding rabbit behavior and employing effective training techniques can lead to a rewarding relationship with your furry companion. Teaching basic commands like "come" and "stay" not only provides mental stimulation for your rabbit but also strengthens the bond between you. By addressing common behavioral issues such as chewing and digging with appropriate solutions, you can create a harmonious environment that caters to your rabbit's natural instincts.

With a focus on positive reinforcement, gentle training methods, and socialization, you can help your rabbit become a well-adjusted, confident pet. Remember that each rabbit is unique, and tailoring your approach to their personality and needs will foster a fulfilling partnership. By investing time and effort into understanding and training your rabbit, you will be rewarded with a loving, loyal companion who brings joy to your life.

CHAPTER 8
ENRICHMENT AND EXERCISE

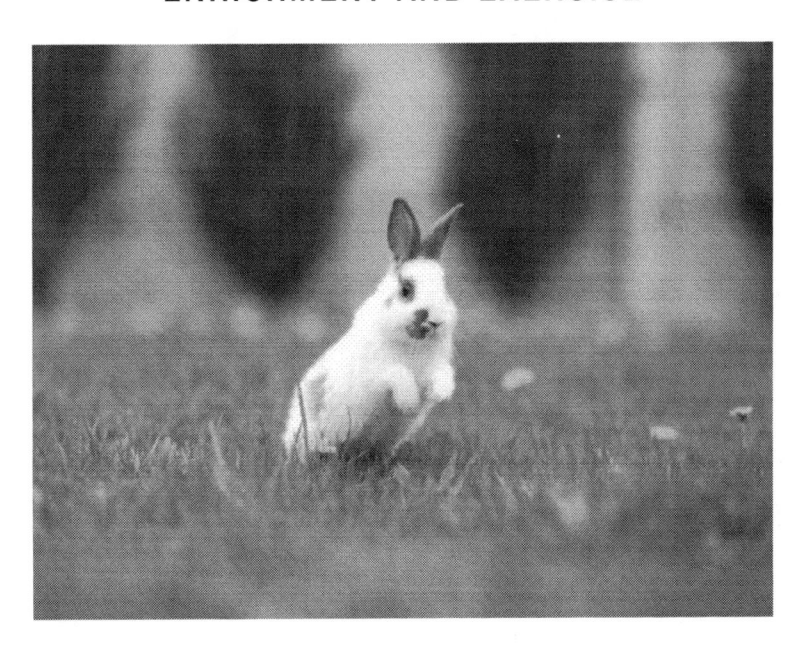

Rabbits are active and intelligent creatures that require both mental and physical stimulation to thrive. Enrichment and exercise are critical components of rabbit care, helping to prevent boredom, mitigate behavioral issues, and promote overall health and well-being. This chapter will discuss the importance of mental and physical stimulation for rabbits, provide ideas for interactive toys and activities, and offer guidance on creating a playtime routine that includes safe outdoor play and bonding activities.

The Importance of Mental and Physical Stimulation and Understanding Rabbit Behavior

1. Natural Instincts: In the wild, rabbits spend much of their time foraging for food, digging, exploring, and interacting with their environment. These natural behaviors are essential for their physical and mental health. Without appropriate stimulation, pet rabbits can become bored, leading to destructive behaviors and stress.

2. Behavioral Benefits: Providing enrichment can help reduce stress, anxiety, and aggression in rabbits. Engaging their minds through play and exploration can also promote healthier behaviors, such as litter box use and social interactions.

Ideas for Interactive Toys and Activities

1. Foraging Toys:

Purpose: Foraging toys encourage rabbits to search for their food, mimicking their natural behavior of scavenging. This not only provides mental stimulation but also slows down their eating, which can aid digestion.

Examples:

Hay Feeder: Use a hay rack or a foraging ball filled with hay and treats, encouraging your rabbit to work for their food.

Puzzle Feeders: Invest in puzzle feeders that require your rabbit to manipulate the toy to access hidden treats.

2. Chew Toys:

Purpose: Chewing is a natural behavior for rabbits, and providing safe chew toys is essential for dental health and mental stimulation.

Examples:

Untreated Wood Chew Toys: Look for toys made from untreated wood, which are safe for rabbits to chew.

Cardboard Boxes: Cardboard is an excellent alternative for chewing and can also be transformed into tunnels or hideouts.

3. Interactive Games:

Purpose: Engaging your rabbit in interactive games can foster bonding and provide physical exercise.

Examples:

Hide and Seek: Hide treats around the room or inside boxes and encourage your rabbit to find them. This stimulates their natural foraging instincts.

Obstacle Course: Set up a simple obstacle course using tunnels, boxes, and safe household items. Guide your rabbit through the course using treats.

4. Tunnels and Hiding Spots:

Purpose: Tunnels and hiding spots provide both physical activity and a sense of security for your rabbit.

Examples:

Commercial Tunnels: Purchase tunnels made specifically for rabbits, or create DIY tunnels using cardboard boxes or PVC pipes.

Hiding Spots: Incorporate hideouts in your rabbit's space, such as small boxes or igloo-shaped shelters where they can retreat when feeling overwhelmed.

5. Social Interaction:

Purpose: Social interaction is vital for your rabbit's mental health. Regular interaction with their human companions or other rabbits can prevent loneliness and boredom.

Examples:

Gentle Petting: Spend time petting and grooming your rabbit, allowing them to bond with you.

Training Sessions: Engage in short training sessions to teach commands or tricks, providing mental stimulation and reinforcing your bond.

Creating a Playtime Routine

Importance of a Structured Routine

1. Predictability: Establishing a playtime routine helps your rabbit understand when to expect interaction and stimulation. This predictability can reduce anxiety and make your rabbit feel more secure in their environment.

2. Physical and Mental Health: Regular playtime ensures that your rabbit receives adequate physical exercise while also stimulating their mind. This can lead to a healthier, happier, and more balanced rabbit.

Safe Outdoor Play

1. Benefits of Outdoor Play:

Variety of Environments: Outdoor play exposes your rabbit to different stimuli, such as grass, leaves, and fresh air. This variety can enhance their natural foraging instincts and provide new experiences.

Physical Activity: Running and hopping in a larger outdoor space allows your rabbit to engage in more vigorous exercise, promoting cardiovascular health and muscle strength.

2. Creating a Safe Outdoor Environment:

Secure Enclosures: Use a secure, enclosed area for outdoor play, such as a rabbit pen or a fenced yard. Ensure that the space is free from potential hazards, such as toxic plants, sharp objects, or other animals that could pose a threat.

Supervision: Always supervise your rabbit during outdoor playtime to prevent escape or injury. Keep an eye on their behavior and ensure they are comfortable in the environment.

3. Exploration and Enrichment:

Foraging Opportunities: Scatter fresh herbs or small pieces of vegetables in the grass for your rabbit to find. This encourages natural foraging behavior and adds an element of excitement to outdoor play.

Interactive Play: Use toys or tunnels designed for outdoor use to engage your rabbit in play. This enhances their experience and keeps them mentally stimulated.

Bonding Activities

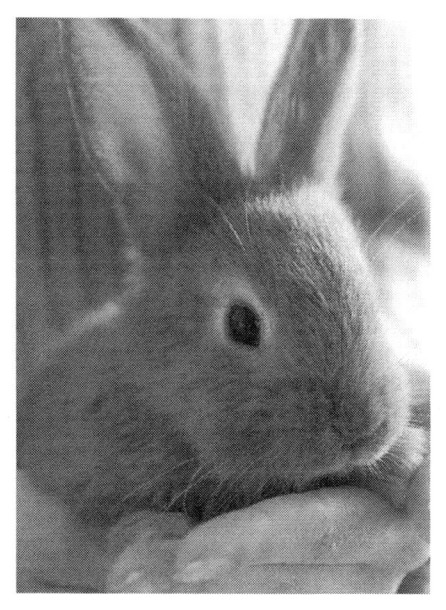

1. Understanding Bonding:

Building a strong bond with your rabbit enhances their trust in you and encourages positive interactions. Bonding activities can help your rabbit feel more secure and engaged in their environment.

2. Daily Interaction:

Playtime: Set aside time each day for interactive play. Use toys, engage in training, or simply sit with your rabbit, allowing them to explore and interact with you at their own pace.

Grooming Sessions: Regular grooming not only helps keep your rabbit's coat healthy but also promotes bonding. Use grooming as an opportunity to provide gentle petting and positive reinforcement.

3. Positive Reinforcement:

Use treats and praise to reinforce good behavior during playtime. This creates a positive association with play and helps build trust between you and your rabbit.

4. Quiet Time:

Spend quiet time with your rabbit, allowing them to relax in your presence. This can be especially beneficial for timid rabbits, helping them to feel comfortable and secure.

Let's explore additional aspects of rabbit enrichment and exercise, including more detailed ideas for activities and toys, the benefits of socialization, and insights into the importance of environmental design for optimal rabbit well-being.

Advanced Enrichment Ideas

1. Interactive Foraging Activities:

DIY Foraging Boxes: Create a foraging box by filling a shallow container with shredded paper or hay and hiding treats within. Encourage your rabbit to dig through the materials to find the hidden goodies.

Hanging Treats: Use a small basket or a mesh bag to hang fresh herbs or vegetables at nose level. This encourages your rabbit to reach and nibble while providing physical and mental stimulation.

2. Sensory Enrichment:

New Scents: Introduce new scents to your rabbit's environment by using safe herbs or toys infused with different materials. For example, using a piece of fleece with a few drops of rabbit-safe essential oils (like chamomile) can provide olfactory stimulation.

Different Textures: Incorporate various textures into your rabbit's space, such as soft fabrics, cardboard, or wooden surfaces. This encourages exploration and adds variety to their environment.

3. Creative Hideouts:

Fort Building: Use cardboard boxes, blankets, and tunnels to create elaborate hideouts or forts. This not only gives your rabbit a place to retreat but also encourages exploration within a safe, enclosed space.

DIY Maze: Construct a maze using cardboard boxes or furniture to create a fun and stimulating environment for your rabbit to explore.

4. Water Play:

While rabbits generally don't swim, they can enjoy supervised play with shallow water. Provide a shallow basin with a few inches of water and floating toys for your rabbit to nudge around. Always supervise closely to ensure safety and comfort.

The Benefits of Socialization

1. Importance of Social Interaction:

Rabbits are social animals that thrive on interaction with humans and other rabbits. Socialization helps them develop confidence and reduces feelings of isolation or stress.

Engaging with your rabbit regularly can lead to better behavior and a stronger bond between you and your pet.

2. Introducing New Friends:

If considering adding another rabbit to your home, ensure both rabbits are spayed/neutered. Introduce them gradually in a neutral, enclosed space to reduce territorial behavior and allow for positive interactions.

3. Group Playtime:

If you have multiple rabbits, allow for supervised group playtime. Monitor their interactions and ensure that they are comfortable and not displaying signs of aggression or fear.

Environmental Design for Rabbit Well-Being

1. Creating a Safe and Stimulating Environment:

Space Requirements: Ensure that your rabbit has enough space to move around freely. A larger enclosure or a designated play area allows for more exploration and exercise.

Vertical Space: Incorporate vertical elements, such as shelves or ramps, to encourage climbing and jumping. Rabbits enjoy exploring different levels and heights.

2. Safe Zones:

Quiet Areas: Provide a quiet retreat where your rabbit can feel safe. This can be a cozy hideaway or a designated corner of their enclosure with soft bedding and minimal disturbances.

Familiar Scents: Use familiar scents, such as blankets or toys that smell like you, to create a calming environment for your rabbit.

3. Variety of Furnishings:

Different Hiding Spots: Offer multiple hiding spots using various materials (e.g., cardboard boxes, fabric tunnels, and wooden huts). This encourages exploration and provides security.

Diverse Flooring: If your rabbit is allowed to roam in a designated space, consider using different flooring materials, such as carpet, tile, or grass, to create a varied texture experience.

Routine and Consistency

1. Establishing a Daily Routine:

Develop a consistent daily routine that includes designated times for feeding, play, social interaction, and quiet time. This helps your rabbit feel secure and understand what to expect throughout the day.

2. Monitoring Behavior:

Observe your rabbit's behavior during playtime to identify preferences and interests. Note which activities they engage with most and adjust your enrichment strategies accordingly.

3. Flexibility:

While routine is important, be flexible in your approach. If your rabbit seems bored or uninterested in certain activities, try introducing new toys or activities to reignite their enthusiasm.

Chapter Summary

Enrichment and exercise are vital aspects of rabbit care that contribute to their overall health and happiness. By providing a variety of interactive toys, engaging activities, and opportunities for social interaction, you can create a stimulating environment that meets your rabbit's physical and mental needs.

Understanding the importance of environmental design, establishing a consistent routine, and fostering socialization will help you nurture a well-adjusted and content rabbit. With patience, creativity, and dedication, you can create a fulfilling and vibrant life for your furry companion, enhancing the bond you share and enriching their daily experiences. Investing time in enriching your rabbit's environment will lead to a happier, healthier, and more engaged pet, allowing you to enjoy the joy and companionship that comes with having a rabbit.

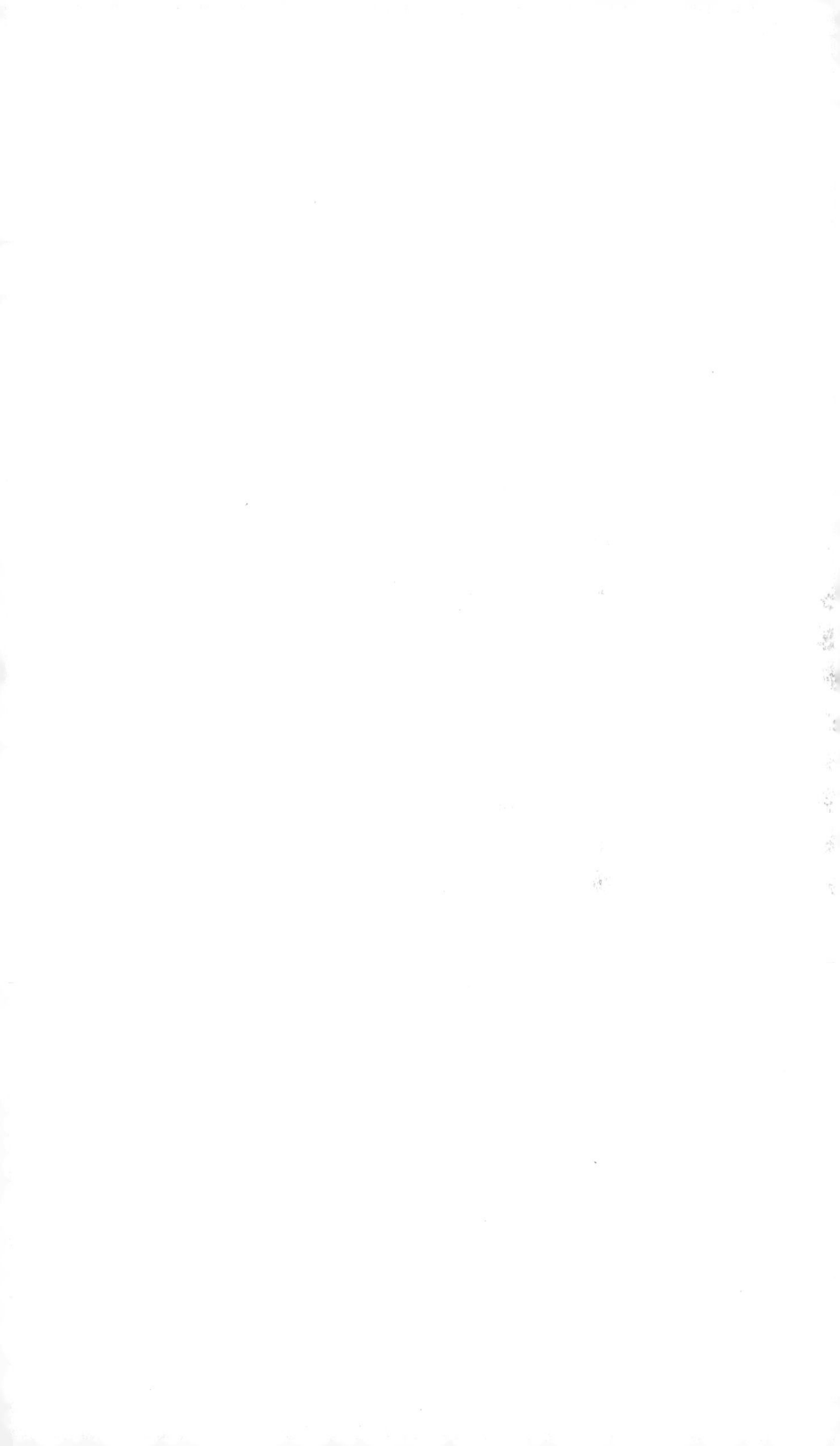

CHAPTER 9
FUN TIPS FOR RABBIT OWNERS

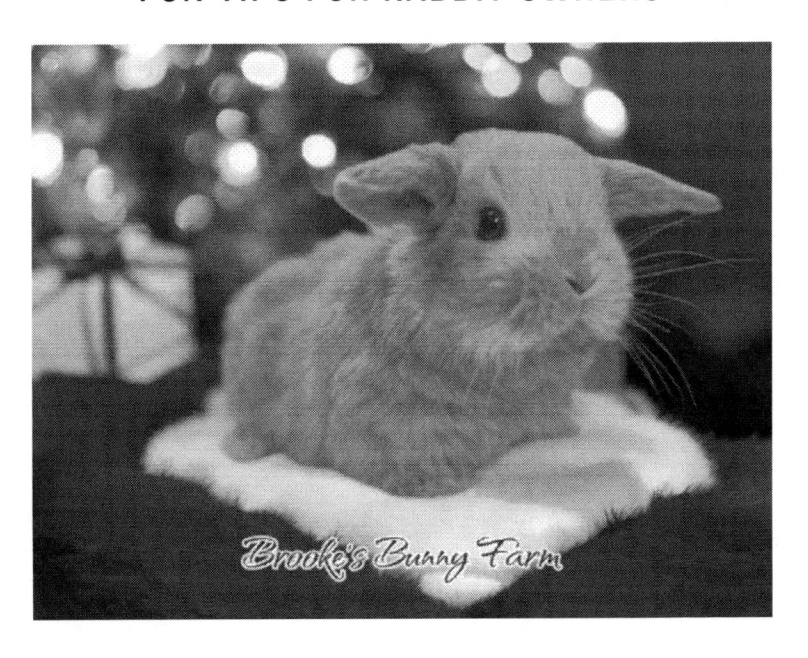

Owning a rabbit can be a delightful experience, filled with unique opportunities for bonding and fun. This chapter will explore creative ways to interact with your rabbit, celebrate special occasions together, and connect with other rabbit owners for support and community.

Creative Ways to Interact and Bond with Your Rabbit

1. Interactive Play Sessions:

Using Toys: Engage your rabbit in interactive play with toys that encourage movement and exploration. Use balls, tunnels, and foraging toys to stimulate their natural instincts. Spend time playing together, allowing your rabbit to explore and learn to trust you.

Training Games: Incorporate training sessions into your bonding time. Teach your rabbit simple commands or tricks using positive reinforcement. This not only strengthens your bond but also promotes mental stimulation.

Obstacle Courses: Design an obstacle course using everyday items like cardboard boxes, tunnels, and chairs. Encourage your rabbit to navigate the course using treats and praise. This not only provides physical exercise but also challenges their mental agility, enhancing their problem-solving skills.

Hide and Seek: Play hide and seek by hiding in different rooms and calling your rabbit. Use treats to encourage them to find you, rewarding them when they do. This interactive game fosters trust and encourages your rabbit to engage with you.

2. Grooming Time:

Bonding Through Grooming: Regular grooming sessions can be a great bonding experience. Use a soft brush to gently groom your rabbit, which mimics the grooming behavior they would experience in the wild. This helps build trust and strengthens your relationship.

Ear and Nail Care: Regularly check your rabbit's ears and nails. While you groom, talk softly to your rabbit to create a calm atmosphere. This interaction can help them feel secure and comfortable.

Regular Grooming Schedule: Establish a grooming routine that includes brushing, nail trimming, and ear cleaning. This not only keeps your rabbit healthy but also builds a strong bond as they become accustomed to being handled gently.

Grooming with Treats: Use treats to make grooming sessions positive. Offer a small treat before you start, and give them another treat after grooming. This creates a positive association with grooming, making it a bonding activity rather than a chore.

3. Exploring Together:

Outdoor Adventures: If your rabbit enjoys being outside, take them on a supervised outdoor adventure. Use a harness and leash or set up a secure pen in the yard. Allow them to explore new sights, sounds, and smells, which can be exciting and enriching for both of you.

Indoor Exploration: Create a safe exploration area indoors where your rabbit can roam freely. Use barriers to block off unsafe areas and provide tunnels and boxes for them to investigate.

Sensory Exploration: Create a sensory experience by introducing different textures and scents. For example, place safe herbs in their space for them to sniff and nibble. Explore new environments together, such as parks, where they can experience the sights and sounds of nature.

Playdates with Supervision: If your rabbit enjoys the company of other rabbits, arrange playdates in a neutral space. Monitor their interactions closely to ensure they are comfortable and positively engaged.

4. Quality Time:

Cuddle Sessions: Some rabbits enjoy cuddling, while others may prefer to sit beside you. Respect your rabbit's comfort level and create a cozy space where they can choose to snuggle or simply be close.

Watch Movies Together: Create a relaxed environment by sitting with your rabbit while watching a movie or reading. Your presence can be comforting for them, and they may enjoy the quiet company.

Interactive Reading: Spend time reading aloud to your rabbit. The sound of your voice can be soothing, and it provides an opportunity to bond without distractions. Your rabbit may enjoy being close to you as you read, creating a calming environment.

Mindful Presence: Simply sitting with your rabbit and observing their behavior can be a bonding experience. Allow them to approach you on their terms, fostering trust and comfort in your presence.

5. Creative Activities:

DIY Projects: Engage in creative projects that include your rabbit. For instance, design a custom play area or create homemade toys together. Involving your rabbit in the process can be a fun bonding experience.

Artistic Expression: Use non-toxic, rabbit-safe materials to create art inspired by your rabbit. You can make paw print art by gently pressing their paw into non-toxic paint and onto paper, creating a memorable keepsake.

DIY Toy Making: Engage your rabbit in creative projects by making toys together. Use safe materials like paper towel rolls, cardboard, and untreated wood to construct various toys. Allow your rabbit to explore the materials as you work.

Bunny Photoshoots: Organize themed photoshoots with props that reflect your rabbit's personality. Use treats to encourage them to pose, capturing adorable moments that celebrate your bond.

Celebrating Special Occasions with Your Rabbit

Ideas for Rabbit-Themed Parties and Events

1. Birthday Celebrations:

Special Treats: Celebrate your rabbit's birthday with special treats. Prepare a small cake made from rabbit-safe ingredients, such as mashed banana and hay, or create a platter of their favorite vegetables and fruits.

Decorations: Use rabbit-themed decorations, such as banners and balloons (make sure they're safe and non-toxic). Set up a cozy area for your rabbit and invite family members to join in the celebration.

Create a Birthday Playlist: Compile a playlist of soft, calming music to play during your rabbit's birthday celebration. This adds a festive atmosphere and can help calm your rabbit during the event.

Special Gifts: Consider gifting your rabbit a new toy or a cozy new bed as a birthday present. Wrap the gift in non-toxic wrapping paper for added excitement, allowing your rabbit to explore and tear open the wrapping.

2. Holidays and Seasonal Events:

Easter Celebrations: Create a bunny-friendly Easter egg hunt using small cardboard boxes or hidden treats around your home. Use rabbit-safe toys or snacks as "eggs" for your rabbit to find.

Halloween Fun: Dress your rabbit in a cute, comfortable costume or create a themed environment with decorations. You can also carve a bunny-shaped pumpkin for added fun.

Christmas Celebrations: Incorporate rabbit-safe decorations, such as garlands made from dried herbs or safe toys hanging from the tree. Consider making a small "stocking" filled with treats for your rabbit to enjoy.

Themed Events: Host a themed event based on your rabbit's personality. For example, if your rabbit is particularly energetic, organize a "bunny Olympics" with fun challenges and obstacle courses.

3. Rabbit Playdates:

If you have friends with rabbits, organize a rabbit playdate. Ensure that all rabbits are spayed/neutered and introduce them in a neutral space. Provide plenty of toys and hiding spots to keep them entertained.

Structured Activities: Plan structured activities for the playdate, such as relay races or treat hunts. This encourages interaction and helps socialize the rabbits in a fun, engaging manner.

Bonding with Owners: Encourage owners to share their experiences and tips while the rabbits play. This fosters friendships between owners as well, creating a supportive environment.

4. Photo Sessions:

Celebrate special occasions by organizing a photoshoot with your rabbit. Use props, costumes, or themed backgrounds to capture adorable moments. This can be a fun way to create lasting memories and share your joy with others.

Themed Costumes: Use costumes that fit the occasion, ensuring they are comfortable and safe for your rabbit. This can add a fun element to your photoshoot while making memorable keepsakes.

Photo Collage: Create a photo collage or scrapbook of your rabbit's milestones and special moments. This can be a great way to reflect on your journey together and celebrate their life.

Community and Resources

Connecting with Other Rabbit Owners and Finding Support

1. Online Communities:

Social Media Groups: Join rabbit-focused groups on platforms like Facebook, Instagram, or Reddit. These groups often share tips, experiences, and resources, allowing you to connect with fellow rabbit enthusiasts.

Forums and Websites: Participate in online forums dedicated to rabbit care. Websites like The House Rabbit Society and RabbitTalk offer valuable information and a space to ask questions and seek advice from seasoned rabbit owners.

Social Media Challenges: Participate in rabbit-themed challenges on platforms like Instagram or TikTok. Sharing your rabbit's antics can connect you with others and allow you to celebrate your pet's personality.

2. Local Rabbit Clubs and Organizations:

Find a Local Club: Many areas have local rabbit clubs or rescue organizations that host events, workshops, and social gatherings. Participating in these groups can provide support, resources, and opportunities to meet other rabbit owners.

Adoption Events: Attend local adoption events or rabbit shows to meet other rabbit owners and learn more about rabbit care. These events often feature vendors and experts who can share valuable insights.

Participate in Events: Attend local rabbit shows, fairs, or educational events organized by clubs. These events often feature workshops, demonstrations, and opportunities to meet other rabbit lovers.

Support Local Rescues: Volunteer or foster for local rabbit rescues. This not only helps the rabbits in need but also connects you with fellow rabbit enthusiasts who share your passion.

3. Veterinary Resources:

Find a Rabbit-Savvy Veterinarian: Building a relationship with a veterinarian who specializes in rabbit care is essential. They can provide guidance on health, nutrition, and general care, ensuring your rabbit remains healthy and happy.

Attend Workshops: Some veterinary clinics and rabbit organizations offer workshops on rabbit care, training, and behavior. Participating in these can enhance your knowledge and help you connect with other rabbit owners. Participating in workshops organized by veterinary clinics or rabbit organizations will help you stay informed about the latest care practices and health information.

4. Volunteer Opportunities:

Rabbit Rescues: Consider volunteering at local rabbit rescues or shelters. This not only helps the rabbits in need but also provides opportunities to learn from experienced caretakers and connect with other rabbit lovers.

Community Events: Participate in community events that promote rabbit awareness and education. Engaging in these activities can broaden your network and provide valuable resources.

Community Involvement: Engage in community outreach programs that promote rabbit awareness. This can include educational presentations at schools or community centers, helping others understand the joys of rabbit ownership.

Organize Fundraisers: Participate in or organize fundraisers to support local rabbit rescues. This helps raise awareness and resources for rabbits in need while connecting you with like-minded individuals.

Chapter Summary

Engaging in unique bonding activities, celebrating special occasions, and fostering connections within a supportive community significantly enrich the experience of rabbit ownership. By dedicating time and creativity to your relationship with your rabbit, you can cultivate a nurturing and joyful environment that benefits both of you.

The strategies and ideas presented in this chapter not only enhance your rabbit's quality of life but also strengthen the bond between you, making your shared journey even more fulfilling. The joy of rabbit ownership is magnified through shared experiences, celebrations, and interactions with fellow rabbit enthusiasts, forming a vibrant community that honors the happiness and affection that rabbits bring into our lives.

By implementing these engaging tips and activities, you can create a rewarding life for your rabbit, characterized by love, laughter, and cherished memories. Whether through interactive play, festive celebrations, or community involvement, the journey of rabbit ownership offers companionship and joy, enriching both your life and that of your rabbit.

CLOSING NOTES FROM THE AUTHOR

Thank you for exploring the world of rabbit ownership through this comprehensive guide. As you have learned in the previous chapters, understanding your rabbit's needs—from their unique behaviors and dietary requirements to their health and wellness—is essential for creating a fulfilling life for both you and your furry companion.

We began by delving into the various rabbit breeds and their characteristics, emphasizing the importance of socialization and companionship in fostering a happy and well-adjusted rabbit. Setting up a rabbit-friendly home, complete with safe living spaces and essential supplies, allows you to provide the best environment for your pet.

Nutrition is a cornerstone of rabbit care, and we highlighted the significance of a balanced diet that includes hay, fresh vegetables, and appropriate pellets. Understanding the basics of litter box training and addressing common challenges ensures a harmonious living situation, while regular veterinary care and preventative health measures keep your rabbit thriving.

Additionally, we explored effective training techniques for teaching basic commands and addressing behavioral issues, which are crucial for enhancing your communication with your rabbit. Enrichment and exercise play vital roles in your rabbit's mental and physical health, and we provided numerous ideas for engaging activities and playtime routines.

Finally, we shared fun tips for rabbit owners, focusing on unique bonding activities, celebrating special occasions, and connecting with a supportive community of fellow rabbit enthusiasts. These elements not only enrich the lives of rabbits but also cultivate joyful and memorable experiences for their owners.

As you embark on your journey with your rabbit, remember that each moment spent together is an opportunity for connection and love. By applying the insights and strategies outlined in this book, you can create a nurturing environment that enhances the quality of life for your rabbit and deepens the bond you share.

May your experience as a rabbit owner be filled with joy, companionship, and countless cherished moments. Thank you for reading, and may you enjoy every hop, cuddle, and adventure with your beloved rabbit!

Best Wishes on your rabbit adventures,
Ryan Warner

Made in the USA
Las Vegas, NV
28 March 2025

a275c6fa-993d-41ba-8af9-5fd20560b28dR02

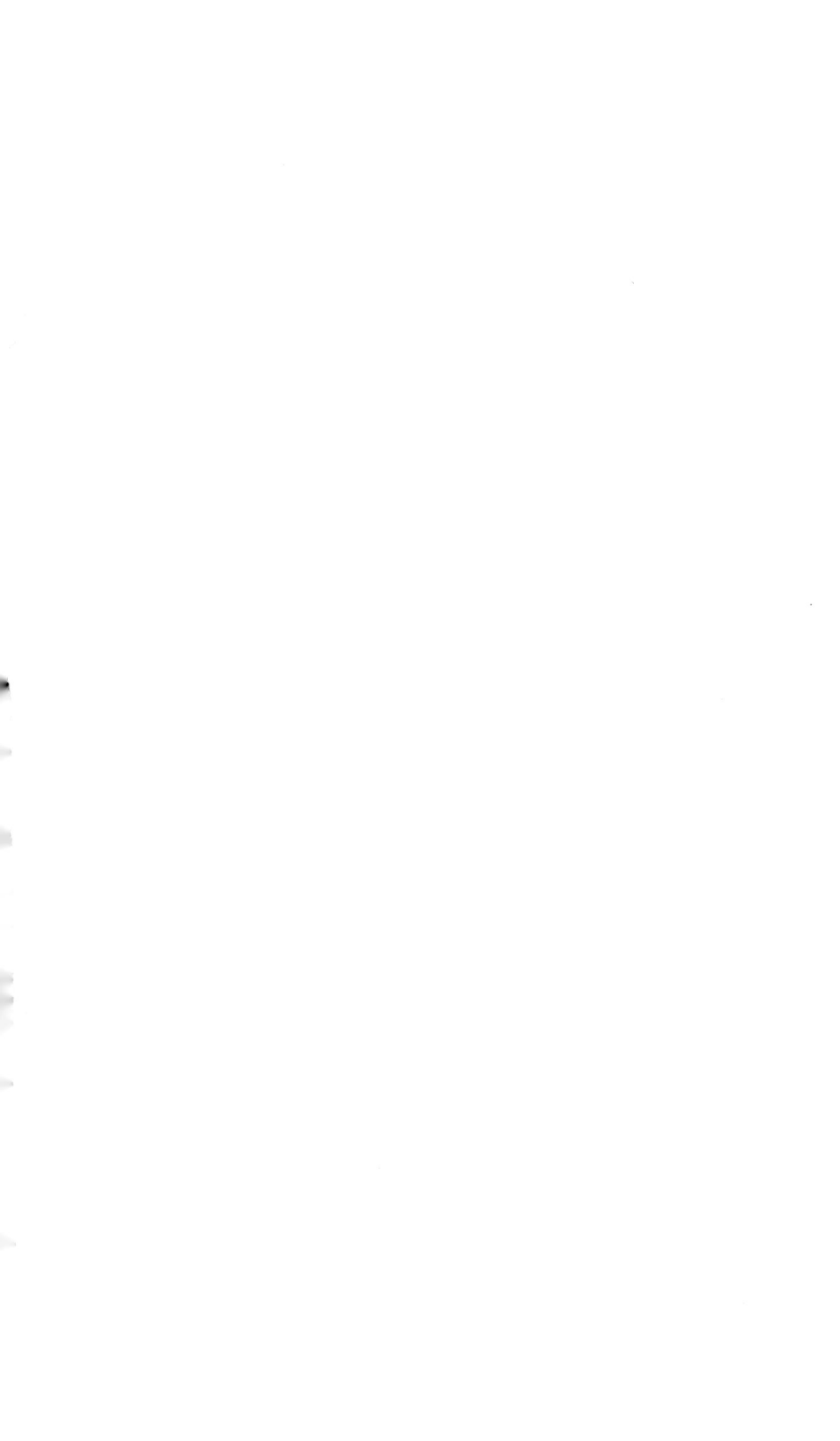

© 1996 by Ruth Davis Williams. All rights reserved.

For information contact:

Heritage House, Publishers
P.O. Box 6135
Lincoln Center, MA 01773
(617) 259-8771

Cover by Catherine F. Meeks

First Printing
Printed in the United States of America
ISBN 1-882063-35-X

Living and Learning

Thirty Years of Wisdom and Advice
from a Prominent Pharmacist

Nellie Davis Poulsen

Edited by Ruth Davis Williams

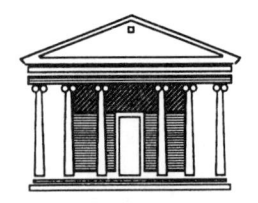

Heritage House, Publishers
Lincoln, Massachusetts

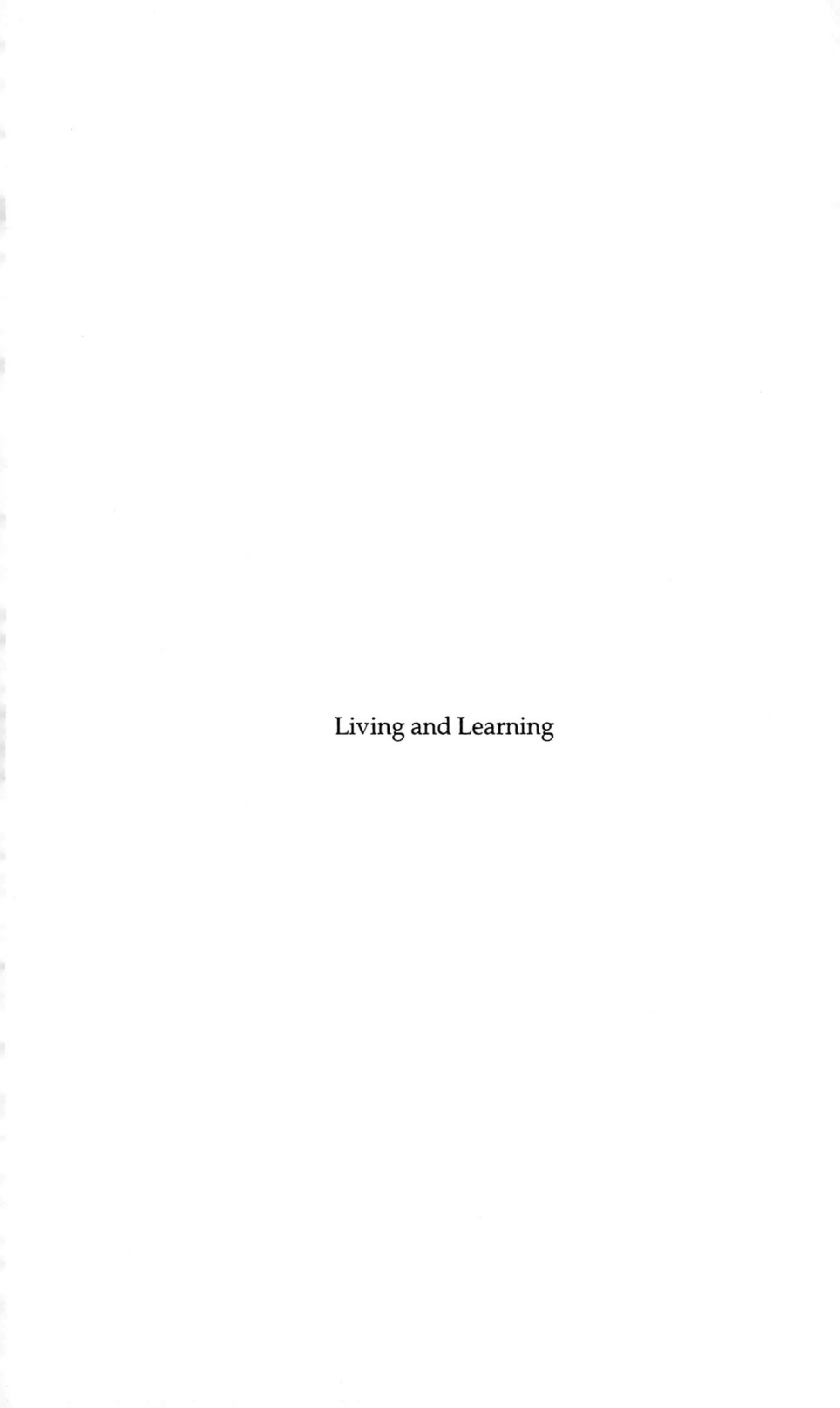

Living and Learning

Contents

Foreword	x
Introduction	xi
The View	1
My Clever Granny	3
Moon Rhyming	5
Pokeweed and Dandelions	6
Licorice	8
Lilies	9
Spring Rain	10
A Gardener's Work	11
Vitamins	13
The Green Season	15
Shamrock	16
Tobasco	17
Shadows	19
Music in the Woods	21
Poison Plants	22
Colchicin	23
Of Mice and Me	24
Sheridan Valley	25
Smile	27
Reward of Using Herbs	28
Pests on Houseplants	29
Cooking with Herbs	31
What Used to Be	35
Mother Nature's Spring	33
Bay Leaves	36
Violets	37
Knitting	38

Foxglove	39
Rosemary	40
Healing Aloe	42
Parsley	43
Good Readers	44
The Miracle of Life	45
Cattails	47
Vitamin B1	48
Sounds of Spring	49
Voices	50
Dandelion	51
Fiddleheads	52
Sage	53
Honey	54
A Snowy Owl	55
Roses	56
Yogurt	57
Vitamin C	58
The Day Is Done	59
Plants' Emotions	61
Mint	62
Six Senses	63
Open Books, Open Doors	64
She's a Lady	65
Vanilla	66
Work and Play	67
Oregano	68
I Like to Paint!	69
Bread	71
Small Things in Life	72
Growing Things	73
There Is Always Music	75
Night Rain	76
Garlic with Hollyhocks	77

Touching Is an Antidote	78
Color Behavior	79
Chervil	80
What Is Beauty?	81
Alfalfa	82
Letter Writing, a Lost Art?	84
Witches Garden	85
Carrots	86
Vitamin	87
Potpourri	88
Plants, Living Together	90
Just Sounds	91
Jewel Weed	93
Medicinal Plants along the Road	94
The Pharmacist	95
Walking and Yoga	97
The Versatile Vinegar	98
Late Summer	99
Geraniums	101
Ambergris	102
Plants Clean Pollution	104
A Summer Morning	105
Herbs Dry and Fresh	107
A Hint of Autumn	108
Being Liberated	109
Magnificent Autumn	110
We Are What We Eat	111
Gardening	112
Old Remedies	113
Talk to Plants	115
Night Sounds	117
Longfellow's Autumn	118
Juniper	120
The Brewhouse	121

Healing with Herbs	123
Walking	124
Irish Moss	125
Michigan Autumn	126
Garlic	127
Seeing Again	128
Morning Gremlins	129
Leeks	130
October	131
Myths and Traditions	133
My Fig Tree	134
Salt	135
The Winds	136
Chocolate	137
Autumn's Beauty	138
An "Old Fashioned" Drug Store	139
Trees for Health and Food	140
Time for Aloneness	141
It Is Autumn	143
Witch Hazel	144
Bald Eagles	144
Our Beautiful World	146
Autumn Tapestries	148
A New Day	149
Dr. Diet, Dr. Quiet and Dr. Merryman	150
Six Herb Vinegar	152
Wild Foods	153
Elderberry	154
Winter Stillness	155
My Music	157
Plants' Feelings	159
Sesame Seeds	160
Beauty of Winter	162
Aloe Vera	166

Aloneness Is Needed	166
Crystallized Flowers	167
Hoarfrost	168
Hobbies	170
Beauty Is Everywhere	171
Power of a Smile	172
"All Is Well"	173
Flowers for Winter	174
Using Our Senses	175
Toad in the Hole	176
Beautiful Music	177
Winter Wonderland	178
Your Work Is You	180
Lavender	181
Early American Herb Recipes	182
Laughter	183
Fairyland	184
No One Listens to Me	186
Beautiful Skin	187
A Smile, a Laugh	188
Freezing Herbs	189
Children	190
Juneberries	191
Vinegar, The Workhorse	192
Beauty in Winter	193
Mistletoe	195
Christmas	197
The Wood Stove	199
Kindness	201
My Dream Harvest	196
A Zest for Life	202
The Boy with the Pipe	205
So, You'd Like to Fill a Prescription!	209
About the Author	213

Foreword

Nellie Poulsen's column in the *Montmorency County Tribune* has added a unique quality to our newspaper. Among the usual news of the day, the local happenings and events, appeared this precious nugget of information and comment that added a deeper perspective. It offers insight into people's lives and their relationship with nature and each other, and lifts the reader above the level on which we live our everyday lives.

Her knowledge of natural herbs and plants reflected something much greater than the usual "how to" column. It portrays Nellie's own view that any person, equipped with knowledge and an insatiable curiosity, can live a self-reliant, productive life in tune with nature and the world.

Nellie came by one day to tell us that she had received a lifetime achievement award from the Michigan Pharmacists Association for her long-time service. She had been one of few women pharmacists and drug store owners through some hard times and satisfying growth times, and it was quite an accomplishment. But the association had printed her name on a standard certificate that described in glowing terms "his" service and "his" dedication. Nellie's flashing eyes were visible in the letter she wrote to accompany that award back to the association. It contained some fine Irish language telling them to either re-write it or do something else with it! A corrected award arrived in short order.

Nellie's association with the Atlanta Art Guild, and the enjoyable time this small group had painting together each Tuesday morning in the Atlanta Library, also enriched those lives, and the lives of all who enjoyed their finished work.

We hope those who read this book enjoy its contents as much as we have enjoyed our association with Nellie. We are indebted to her for making our small town newspaper something extra special to our readers for many, many years.

Tom and Carol Young
Montmorency County Tribune

Introduction

My Mother the Writer
When I was in Pharmacy School at Wayne University, I had to write a biography about a parent in English class. I went to school full time and worked forty-eight hours in the drug store. There was no time to think and write. I kept asking mother about her life and finally she said "I will write it; you go and deliver the prescription to a customer." When I got back she had it written—on wrapping paper! I turned it in the next day and got an "E," which meant failing, not excellent! So the writer of two novels and several short stories didn't pass that test. And the professor was a very good customer of ours—always sick!

My Mother the Cook
After I was married, living in Cambridge, Mother called me one Sunday morning. "Ruth, how do you peel an egg for deviled eggs?" I told her and she called back and said it had green around the yolk, and "What should I do now?" Being sassy, I said put lots of parsley in it. It was a hit, and from that day on she put parsley in everything!

My Mother the Mother
I made many deliveries at night, and had my driver's license at fourteen. Every time I went out any distance, a car would follow me and park about a block away and turn off the lights. I was always scared. Many years later she told me she called the police to follow me and see that no harm came to me. Wish I had known then!

My Mother the Pharmacist
The Depression days hit "the corner drug store" very hard all over the country, but she survived by being kind to everyone. She never said NO if a person couldn't pay. She did a lot of

counter prescribing in those days for people who couldn't pay a doctor. She had a good reputation with the doctors. They would call her for information on new drugs. She always had time to listen to the "detail men" who gave the druggists information on new medicines his company had to offer. She had a world of medical information in her head and knew where to find it. Mother and I had a great relationship. We learned from each other. We were friends.

Ruth Davis Williams

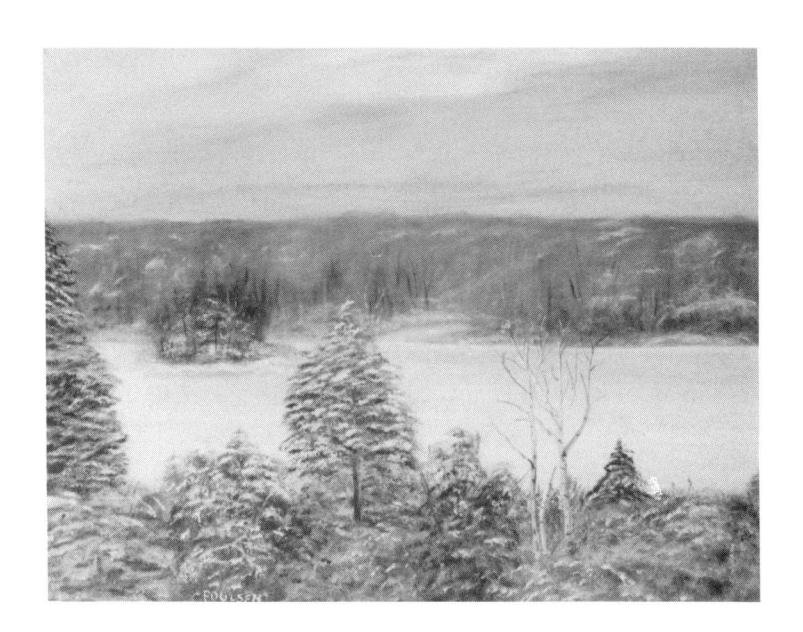

The View

Our home is on a hill above a lake and we are privileged to observe some rather wonderful things at times. Eagles soaring and sailing across the sky, or hurrying to their nesting places up the river. Beautifully feathered hawks with sharp eyes peering through the treetops in quest for bird's nests. Fantastic sunsets with colors that stir the senses and make one feel very humble. Stars that stud the dark-blue curtain of night and sometimes shower a few meteorites across the sky. Sunrise turning the hills scarlet and making magic of early-morning mist.

A few evenings ago, I was standing outside on the porch looking into the turbulent clouds that presaged a storm. There was ominous beauty in the vast-moving billows of grey, a beauty that sent shivers down my spine. In the distance I heard the sound of geese coming in a straight line down the lake. Presently two huge flocks converted overhead, their cry, a pitiful exhausted sound, like that of weary children. Evidently scouts had come ahead of the flock, for they wheeled round and round until assured it was safe to land. Then slowly, blue-grey wings fluttered downwards into the darkened water and the honking subsided into sleepy, contented murmurings.

This April morning I can see soft greens across the hill, and I am thankful that I am privileged to once more witness the miracle of returning life. To see the tender green of plants you were sure had been killed by winter frost; to hear again the song of robins and the raucous croak of the first frogs, and the loud, happy honking heralding the departure of the migrating birds. Another day is born!

――― ❖ ―――

My Clever Granny

My Granny had it made. It's a fact I have been pondering on for half an hour or so. I firmly believe she had more natural gumption than I'll ever have. She had all the cleverness, craftiness, cunning and charm of the Irish with a knowhow that really mattered. She ate well, slept with a clear conscience, indulged in good laughs whenever the mood took her and she had more knowledge about crude drugs than I'll ever be able to stow in my noodle.

Granny was a widow when a very young woman. She was without benefit of social security, pensions, or a nest egg salvaged from the days of marriage, yet I never heard her complain. Living in a remote village without benefit of doctor or nurse, she yet managed to doctor the whole community, ring the church bell for vesper services, keep the communion plate in a highly polished state and arrange for burial places for the dead. Because of her glorious flower garden she would, for a given sum, arrange to plant flowers on the graves of the dear departed, provided the relatives lived too far away to do the job themselves.

I well remember an occasion when a canny Scotsman arranged with Granny to plant the grave of his mother. All was well 'til Granny bounced the sovereign he left with her on the kitchen hearth. The ring was dull, but the crop of dandelions on the MacDonald burial plot was golden.

She was without competition in any of the various jobs she undertook, but I wish I had even a small amount of her courage. I'd like some of her advice and I wish I had been blessed with some of her canny humor and aplomb. She gave vent to her imagination without restraint, and because of her knowledge, she was greatly beloved by the villagers. I can still see her coming down the hillside with her apron full of wood betony, yarrow and chamomile and I shudder in retrospect as I again smell the concoction she brewed from these herbs for the coughs and colds of the local folk.

She gathered tranquility from the woods she tramped and it was all reflected in the blue of her eyes. Her body was fragrant with the oil she pressed from lavender, begamot and stock. Her heart was content because of the many kindnesses she performed through her homeopathic use of herbs. Yes, Granny had it made. Her heart ruled her life and no man had the temerity to show her which way to go.

❖

Moon Rhyming

Last night the moon was full. I know that tides run high, dogs howl, coyotes set up a racket, and witches prowl when the moon is full. What I can't understand is why I can't sleep when that heavenly body shines through my window. There could be a bit of lunacy in me, but I challenge anyone else to suggest such a possibility. I just lie there, count my blessings and discard a few things not in the blessing category; then I begin to compose verses, trying to make unrhymable words rhyme.

My Irish Granny had her own special remedy for coping with full moon sleepless nights. She filled a good-sized mug with porter, pushed the poker into the fire and when it was red hot plunged it into the porter and leisurely, and with apparent pleasure, sipped the concoction. She assured us that the night of the full moon was the only time she used the warm porter, and of course, we believed her.

People have different methods of dealing with sleeplessness. Some count sheep, while many just take a sleeping pill. I leave sheep alone for I had to help my grandfather during sheep-shearing as a child. I'll stick to my rhyming.

When I lived on the south coast of England, it wasn't necessary to look at an almanac to find out what the moon was up to. The tides rolled far into the caves and the waves were high and most people were a bit edgy. I haven't noticed any appreciable difference in my sweet disposition, although some folk might disagree, but I do need sleep. I could get up and start cleaning house, bake a cake, read a book or prepare a witches brew, but I'm hooked on rhyming. Moon rhyming is easy. There's a room, loon, tune, loom etc. but what the dickens rhymes with lunacy? Perhaps I'll get over this phobia by the time I reach a sensible age, but I'll take a new moon any old night.

❖

Poke Weed and Dandelions

Despite the inclement weather, there are many greenings pushing through the moist earth. The young shoots of pokeweed are flourishing in the rich soil outside the compost bins. This plant, which many people call poke salad has leaves shaped like a lance head. The poke must be gathered when the shoots are no higher than three to four inches. Many southerners fry these young shoots, but they are particularly delicious just boiled and eaten as a vegetable. Cook in boiling water for ten minutes, discard the water, and either steam or boil again until the leaves are tender. The bitter principle is discarded with the first water and what is left is similar in taste to asparagus. The young shoots can also be pickled.

The precious dandelion, while loath to face the cool mornings, is showing young, succulent leaves. If you can spare some from your salads, try a few recipes. Tear the leaves of the young plant and toss with hot vinegar sweetened with a little sugar and flavored with a scraping of fresh onion. Cook a few slices of bacon until crisp and add to the wilted leaves. Garnish with hard boiled eggs and enjoy! Or steam the young leaves, add butter and pepper, just that! Why we disdain this plant and delegate it to the weed department, is because we haven't learned, as did our ancestors, to use it to ward off sicknesses caused by lack of vitamins A and C.

If there is a beverage as fine as dandelion wine as my Granny made it, I don't know what it could be. Think of the sunshine stored in those golden blossoms.

I hope you can recognize the beautiful Jerusalem artichoke plant which grows tall and has blossoms like the sunflower. They can be found along the roadside in some places. Mine have taken over the outer part of the garden, where the tubers remain all winter. In spring they are most welcome. Sliced thinly in a salad, served as a snack with a good dip, or just plain boiled. Try steaming them and serve with herbed butter. Dip large slices in egg and breadcrumbs and fry them and do remember this tuber is highly recommended for diabetics.

"And God said: 'Behold, I have given you every herb bearing seed, which is upon the face of the Earth. . . to you it shall be meat.'" — Genesis.

❖

Licorice

Do you remember the licorice stick that left our tongues black but tasted so good? And do you curl up your nose as you recall being dosed with licorice powder in early spring? That wasn't too enjoyable, and, since my Granny always mixed the powder in milk, I've had little respect for milk ever since. Most people think that all drugs are synthetically prepared, but that is not the case. As we add up all the prescription drugs derived from natural sources, they account for almost 50 percent of the ingredients.

Licorice, or, as some folk call it, sweet wood, is known to pharmacy as Glycyrrhiza and is grown in many parts of the world. It is native from Southern Europe to Pakistan and Northern India, but it is also grown in England, Belgium and France. Licorice is fifty times sweeter than glucose, and the addition of one pound of licorice will double the sweetness of 100 pounds of sugar. The plant may be grown from seed, but the usual method is by dividing the root. It grows best in rich, moist soil, but it is necessary that the late summer is hot and dry in order to obtain good ripe pods and healthy root system.

Glycyrrhiza increases fluid and plasma in the body and it is often given to desert troops to prevent extreme thirst on low water intake. It is a common ingredient in cough syrups and cough drops, not only for its flavor but also for its demulcent properties and anti-inflammatory action. A thick syrup of water and licorice is often prescribed for stomach and duodenal ulcers but it will often cause edema and hypertension.

In India, licorice powder is mixed with fat and honey and is applied to cuts and wounds. The United States imports 27,000 tons of licorice root each year.

Why did I write about licorice? I saw a small boy sucking on a stick of the black stuff. It ran down his shirt front and I wondered what washing powder his mother would be using.

❖

Lilies

This morning my thoughts are on lilies, perhaps because I have a very beautiful white amaryllis blooming on the windowsill and this plant belongs to the lily family.

Lilies have an old history, perhaps the oldest of all flowers. There is a legend which says the lily sprang from the tears of Eve when she was forced to leave the Garden of Eden. A Korean legend tells of a hermit who found a tiger wounded and in pain. He removed an arrow from its paw and the animal became his inseparable companion. When the tiger died, they discovered it had begged to be buried next to its rescuer and friend, and from that mound of earth grew a lily that was striped, the tiger lily.

Then, when the hermit was drowned, the lilies spread all over the earth in an attempt to find him. No flower is as generally known and accepted as is the lily. In India, China, Egypt and Japan it is accepted as a symbol of fruitfulness. To the Japanese the lilies were the symbol of peace and war, the white lily for peace and the tiger lily for war.

Among Christian nations the lily stands for purity and chastity. It is a symbol of resurrection and of Easter. It has been said that the original Madonna lily was yellow, but when the Virgin held it in her hands, it became white. In England it was believed that anyone who put their nose too near a tiger lily would become freckled, and anyone daring to tread on one of these flowers would certainly be capable of crushing the purity of the woman in the house.

At one time lilies were used in various treatments. When the roots were ground up and mixed with honey, they would glue together severed muscles. Leaves and roots were used for burns and scalds and to dissolve tumors. In Hungary it is believed that on the spot where an innocent person has been executed, a clump of yellow lilies will spring up.

Guess I'll go and ask my lily if she approves of what I have just written.

Spring Rain

There are all kinds of rain, some accompanied by blustery, cold gales interspersed with hail which makes a good fire feel very comforting. However, about this time of year, God turns over the coin and sends us spring rain. Soft, caressing, warm.

To walk through the woods when the earth opens her mouth to the gentleness of this moisture, to feel the playful patter of raindrops on your upturned face—this is happiness.

Shining leaves of hepatica and wintergreen push aside the leaf-mold of the woods floor and the tightly folded buds of spring beauties, and trailing arbutus make a timid appearance through the cold coverings of winter.

There's a new note in birdland and a merry sound to the river water full to overflowing with the melting snows of April.

Sap runs freely down the trunks of sugar bush and I gather some on the tip of my finger and wish for pancakes and maple candy.

The wings of a chickadee flip through my hair and I swear that bird laughed with glee! A gentle breeze shakes the wetness from pine trees as I walk the last half mile home.

I feel refreshed, renewed, and very thankful to be able to enjoy spring rain.

❖

A Gardener's Work

A gardener works hard and has many frustrations for the privilege of harvesting a few fresh vegetables and enjoying the beauty of blooming flower beds for a few brief weeks each year.

We plant seeds. Some grow, some don't. Have you ever watched with joy as carrot, cucumber and squash pushed their precious green through the earth, even though you were told it was too early to plant seeds? And have you ever experienced the disappointment at seeing the result of the night's frost?

I planted four flats of flowers last week and pridefully contemplated my day's work. Had I been a weeping female I might have indulged in a few tears next morning when I beheld the power of a 28 degree temperature.

But Mother Nature isn't the only one who enjoys playing tricks on us gardeners. The animal kingdom supplies a fair amount of nuisance material in the form of moles, rabbits and woodchucks. Grass is not their idea of gourmet dining. More succulent are peas, lettuce, and asparagus tips.

However, I have an exterminator, who, when allowed to enter the garden, scares the bejabbers out of rabbits and woodchucks, while he kills the moles. It costs an extra can of Alpo, but what exterminator works for nothing. Why, when strawberries ripen, does a chipmunk who manages to get his body through the smallest hole in the fence, decide to taste a small portion of many berries instead of settling for one or two whole ones? My four-footed animal controller could handle the situation, but the damage four feet could do to the strawberries far outweighs the chippy's small mouth activity.

Then there's the matter of bees. Well it's not really matter—it's unpredictability. Why should they be around when I'm weeding and dine on my body when so many plants need pollinating? And for heavens sake, where do slugs, potato bugs and beetles hide until my garden begins to grow?

Frustrated, discouraged and determined to make this the last year I'll pay attention to seed catalogues. You bet your bottom dollar. I've had it!

P. S. I wonder when the catalogues will come next year?—January is a good month!

Vitamins

As I swallowed my vitamins this morning, my thoughts went back to my Granny. "Eat all of it," she would say when we were fortunate enough to have an orange, and "all of it" meant the peel as well as the fruit. I used to wonder why, when I cried with growing pains, Granny gave me a handful of rose hips which she gathered and dried every fall.

Today I take vitamins, although for years doctors have denounced vitamins as unnecessary if enough fruits and vegetables are eaten. Now, thanks to new research, more and more scientists suspect that traditional medical views of vitamins and minerals have been too limited, and that they play a more complex role in assuring optimal health than previously thought.

Here are a few of the helpful tips I have read, and tried. Vitamin E may turn out to be helpful in preventing free radicals from injuring the heart. Research on more than 87,000 women in a famous hospital, indicated that women with a high intake of vitamin E had 36 percent less heart disease than was previously known. Vitamin E also seems to boost the immune system in healthy old people. One of the most important vitamins, however, seems to be beta carotene, a complex deep-orange compound naturally abundant in sweet potatoes, carrots and cantaloupes. *Just don't take overdoses.*

Nutritionists and doctors agree that everyone's basic needs could be met by eating a diet rich in vegetables and fruits. Just how many people are even able to come close to what is recommended: three to five servings daily of vegetables; two to four of fruit; two to three of milk, yogurt and cheese; and two to three of meat, eggs, poultry and fish? It is found that a mere nine percent of adults consume five servings of fruits and vegetables.

New findings about vitamin C are proving to be invaluable, even though we have long known that this vitamin, if deficient in our diet will not help our shortness of breath, swollen or painful joints, anemia and slow healing of wounds. One of the latest reports find a lack of vitamin C causes breaks in the capillary walls.

Fortunately, vitamins promise to unfold as one of the great and hopeful health stories of our day.

❖

The Green Season

Have you ever contemplated the miracle of green? All winter the snow has been piled high on my herb garden, but as I brushed away the debris this morning, there was the delicate green of hoarhound, balm, chervil, parsley and the dark tips of orange mint. I wondered which herbs my Granny would have poured into my ailing body last week had she been alive. In retrospect, I tasted the brew of feverfew, pennyroyal and hoarhound and remembered the word I always used to describe the taste of such decoctions. EVIL! It was my favorite expression during the cold, cough, fever season. And always my Granny's glib rejoinder; "honi soit qui mal y pense." Occasionally the reprimand was softened with a few tender words in Gaelic.

The miracle of green season also brought wonderful fresh foods: nettles, lightly cooked, chopped and mixed with a little flour, butter and cream. Or nettle soup with a good veal or beef bone for base stock. Ginger beer made from nettles and lemons. Nettles! You say, "Those stinging things!" Put on some good gloves and gather all you can, for here is an herb that is heavy with many essential vitamins. Nettle pudding, not a dessert, was one of the favorite spring dishes, chopped up with cabbage and beef and a little finely chopped suet. Season well with pepper and salt and steam until cooked. Sounds awful? Try it and change your mind.

There seems to be an influx of various types of herb teas on the market today—soft, pleasant beverages made to replace soft drinks. But the best drink I can remember was the Spring Ale my Granny made. Three quarts of nettles; one of dandelion leaves. Boil gently with two gallons of water to which has been added two sliced lemons and an ounce of ginger-root. Strain and add two cups of sugar. When lukewarm stir in a cake of yeast which has been dissolved in a little warm water. Bottle immediately and cap tightly. Refrigerate before opening.

❖

Shamrock

For many years I have had a shamrock plant in the house. I love the bright little white flowers and the way in which the plant folds up its bright green leaves at night, slowly opening them when the sun comes up. A shamrock I have had for many years decided a year ago that it needed a long rest. I missed it. On St. Patrick's day a dear friend presented me with a beautiful plant, and the house is again a home!

The three petalled shamrock has become the symbol of a race, as the pale leaf of Canada or the fleur-de-lis of France. But what is the shamrock? Ask any Irishman and he will probably tell you that it is a non-flowering plant that grows only in Ireland. And he will tell you how St. Patrick used the shamrock to preach the trinity when he came to convert Ireland to Christianity in the fifth century.

In the late 19th century the Irish naturalist Nathaniel Colgan undertook to unravel the botanical mystery of the shamrock. The investigation revealed a curious history for the little plant.

According to Colgan, the word "shamrock" first appears in literature in Edmond Campion's *History of Ireland,* published in 1571. Campion asserts that the plant is used as food for the poor Irish. For the next century every reference to the shamrock presents the plant solely as a breadstuff or food-herb of the Irish, so used probably only in times of famine or scarcity of grain. In 1680 an Oxford physician attributed the strength and agility of the Irish to their shamrock diet. Now we are told that all of the plants identified as the "true shamrock" are as common over western Europe as in Ireland. If St. Patrick used the sweet little shamrock of Ireland to preach the Trinity there is no evidence of this event.

Well, I'll go see if my dear shamrock needs a little nourishment.

❖

Tabasco

On those rare days when we are fortunate enough to have shrimp cocktail before dinner, my husband makes the sauce and must always have a few drops of Tabasco. Curiosity led me to look up the history of this necessary-for-shrimp-cocktail ingredient, and this is what I discovered.

The year was 1848 and the Mexican War had ended and, finding the warm, sunny country to their liking, many American soldiers stayed in Mexico. One, known only by the name of Gleason, traveled south from Mexico City and settled there. Later, longing for his own country, he sailed for New Orleans. There, he ran into an old acquaintance, Mr. Edmund McIlhenny. Before the two parted, Gleason gave his friend a handful of dried pepper pods he had brought back from southern Mexico. "You will find," he said, "that these will add exceptional flavor to your food."

Mr. McIlhenny found that his friend had not exaggerated, for the peppers possessed an unusual flavor. He saved some seeds and planted them in the garden of his father-in-law at Avery Island. Before long, family and close friends were treated to the results of a variety of culinary experiments made by Edmund McIlhenny with these amazing peppers.

During the War between the States the Averys and the McIlhennys were forced to leave their homes on Avery Island. After the conflict was over they returned, and Mr. McIlhenny discovered that a number of the pepper plants still flourished. Using these peppers, he experimented anew. His efforts produced one exceptionally exciting red pepper sauce that friends soon referred to as "that wonderful sauce Mr. McIlhenny makes."

Among these friends was General Hazard, Federal Administrator for South Louisiana. On one of his trips north, General Hazard took along several bottles of the sauce for his family and friends. Among them was his brother, Mr. E. C. Hazard of New York, a man who owned one of the largest wholesale grocery houses in America. He was so enthusiastic that he ordered regular shipments to be made to New York.

Next a name was needed, and a fanciful one was selected: Tabasco an Indian word meaning "land where the soil is humid." This aptly describes the small area where the peppers grow best. Since 1868 this word "Tabasco" has been used as the exclusive trademark of the pepper sauce for it is treated like fine wine.

Try a few drops in marinades, gravies, eggs, chicken, meats, and, of course, on those special days when shrimp cocktail is on the menu.

❖

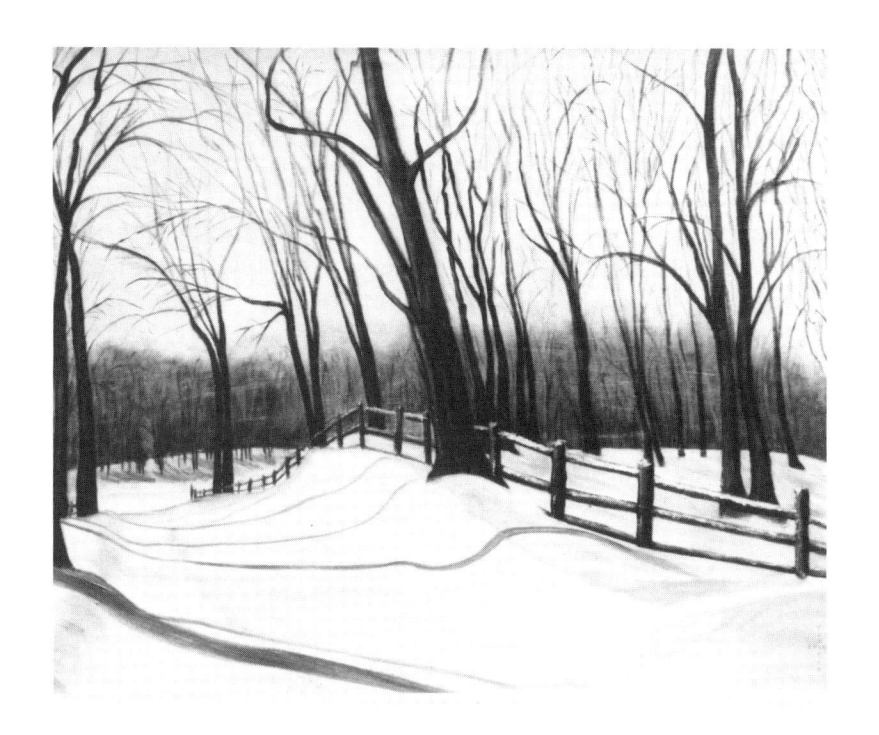

Shadows

A few days ago I was discussing with an artist friend the value of shadows. Shadows may impress one as a rather uninviting field of study, but there are some very interesting facts to be observed in shadows.

It is generally agreed that the most charming of shadows, are tree shadows, sometimes called "shadow lace." The finest quality of the "lacework" is to be seen on the snow in winter when the trees are bare of foliage. Strange as it may seem the beauty of landscape bathed in sunlight and sprinkled with shadows, has been recognized by art only a comparatively short time—all within the last century.

One of the most beautiful effects in music is the increase and diminishing of a tone by imperceptible graduations. And so it is in nature's art. The graduation from light to shadow and vice versa is what creates beauty. The shadows over a distant landscape, reflect the color of the sky and clouds above them so completely that the local color is lost. The bluest of shadows is generally seen upon snow under the intense blue of a winter's sky.

Some artists paint all their pictures in a high key as if they lived in a world of eternal sunshine. Rembrandt immersed everything in a bath of shadow, plunging into even the light itself. He surrounded centers of light with waves of darkness, and his darkness is always transparent. You can peer into it and discover half-concealed forms. Everything provokes curiosity; there is mystery, and it also acts upon the mind so that the real and imaginary become mingled.

To see and understand how charming shadows can be, look over some of the dark and shadowy things in life for their will always be something bright and cheerful beside them.

❖

Music in the Woods

Believe it or not—spring is here. I counted eleven robins and scores of finches this morning. Our snowdrops and crocus are in bloom, and, if I scraped away leaves to look for early dandelion, it's because I'm an optimist. Yes! There are pussy willows and the chipmunks have come out of hibernation, and if I can't see nightcrawlers in the lawn, it's just because my sight is not too good. But they are there!

Forsythia, apple blossom and lilac branches are blooming in the house wafting a fine fragrance across the room, and of course, that is a sure sign that spring is here.

Oh yea! I have seen three flocks of Canada geese winging their way northward ignoring the bald eagle gliding with consummate grace above the lake.

Hepatica leaves are pushing aside the sodden plants of last year and bees are buzzing around where they shouldn't. I've planted seeds indoors and if they damp off, I'll not complain for I've had fun trying. The Easter cactus who thought Easter too early for it to make an effort to bloom, has condescended to vie for importance with the Easter lily my beloved bought me.

The lake speaks in baritone cadences which precedes the breaking up of the ice, and a blue heron stands over a break in the ice, one leg on each side of the water, peering with narcissistic intentness into the dark water. There's a singing sound in the wind and I listen for a melody. My husband said I'm fey to even think such things, then I begin to discourse on the radio waves which surely travel through the air, but I finally admit I know nothing about such things.

But I still hear music in the woods. *"Came the Spring with all its splendor, all its birds and all its blossoms, all its flowers and leaves and grasses."* —Longfellow.

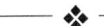

❖

Poison Plants

In the early part of each year, pharmacists are asked to take part in preventing poisoning. We have focused attention on household poisons. However, I wonder if we are all aware of the poison in some of the plants and flowers we grow and gather for decorating our homes. So many of our beautiful plants are poisonous and we should be aware of having them within reach of an inquisitive child.

The lovely Jerusalem Cherry, its bright red fruits a joyful sight on a cold, winter day, is one plant to put beyond the reach of children. And the Winter Crocus, Poinsettia, be it red, pink or cream, contains poisonous juice. Juice from the Deiffenbachia will render the most talkative person mute if the least bit of leaf comes in contact with the tongue. (Please don't get any naughty ideas.) Remember when we indulged in a sprig of mistletoe at Christmastime? You hoped that young lad your mother had invited for dinner would see it suspended from the beam and take the hint? And when the shy, young lug ignored the gesture, didn't you regret spending the money? I wonder if the reason for hanging it out of reach, was because mistletoe is so poisonous?

So many "plants of the field" should be avoided: Jimson Weed, Canadian Thistle, Field Bindweed, Devil's Trumpet and Loco Weed. No one needs to be reminded of poison ivy and sumac. And yet, some poisonous plants are not wholly bad. Certain ones destroy insect pests; and many of them give us valuable drugs such as Aconite, Atropine, Digitalis, Cocaine, Ipecac, Quinine and Strychnine. Then we have tomato, potato, rhubarb and eggplant, all of which are good vegetables, but whose leaves contain a poisonous substance. So does a green potato that has been exposed to light.

I can't imagine a home without flowers; just take precautions.

❖

Colchicin

One of my friends just informed me he was taking Colchicin for gout, and I am about to order Fall Crocus from the nursery. So why do I make associations between gout and Crocus?

The Autumn Crocus belongs to the lily family. It is often called meadow saffron. The corm has numerous fibrous roots and when cut it smells like radishes. The blooms are lavender to light pink and are a joyous sight in Fall when the rest of the flowers begin to fade. The Autumn Crocus is native to grassy meadows, woods and riverbanks in Ireland, England and Denmark. The main ingredient of this beautiful flower is Colchicin, widely used as a remedy for gout, rheumatism, arthritis, dropsy and gonorrhea.

This plant was well known to the ancient Greeks and Romans and the corm was included in the British Pharmacopoeia for many years. Because Colchicin arrests cellular mitosis it was hoped it might be of benefit in cancer therapy, but it is entirely too toxic for such use. All parts of the plant are poisonous, but so are all parts of the regular crocus we welcome with such joy in spring.

The Autumn Crocus looks so much like an onion it is often mistaken for such and people have often died from ingesting this corm so like a vegetable. Prolonged use of Colchicin will cause anemia, neuritis and loss of hair.

There are so many plants which have played an important part in medicine for many generations, plants which still furnish the ingredients of numerous prescriptions and over-the-counter drugs. It is good to know a little something about these plants which can heal, but if abused, can also kill.

❖

Of Mice and Me

Mice! I hate 'em. I'll even admit I'm afraid of them. It all began when I was a small six-year-old. I was taking a bath, when a mouse appeared on the edge of the bathtub. In terror, I jumped out of the tub and ran through the house seeking help. Had my parents been alive they would have understood and comforted me, but instead, I was severely punished for indecent exposure! I hate mice!

My next vivid encounter was with the critters when I was very pregnant. I opened a cupboard door and a mouse jumped on to my tummy. I fainted. If you have never turned down your bed only to find a mouse under your nighty, you have never known the panic I felt one night after a long day's work in the drugstore. I slept for weeks without a nightgown and on the wrong side of the bed. One quiet afternoon in the drug store, my peace of mind was shattered when a mouse ran across the prescription desk. In desperation, I called my husband and asked if he would bring some mouse traps. Fifteen minutes later he walked into the store, carrying in his arms our purring, contented tomcat!

Perhaps the most severe scolding I ever had in my life was from my daughter. We had had a hold-up in the drug store, which was enough annoyance for one day, but as I opened the door to the living room that night, a mouse ran across the floor right at my feet. Naturally, I jumped on the nearest table. My daughter, Ruth, wearing the look of a scolding teacher remarked, "My mother! She can stand up to two gun-toting gangsters and yet she's afraid of a mouse." The critters have no respect for the body of a person.

Oh well! The mouse that was foolish enough to get into a trap in our living room last week, was carefully picked up with a pair of very *long* tongs, and I flung mouse and trap as far outdoors as possible. I'm really getting quite brave.

I wonder why God, after making big animals like elephants, lions and horses, took the trouble to make a mouse. Perhaps He had a bad day. We all get 'em.

❖

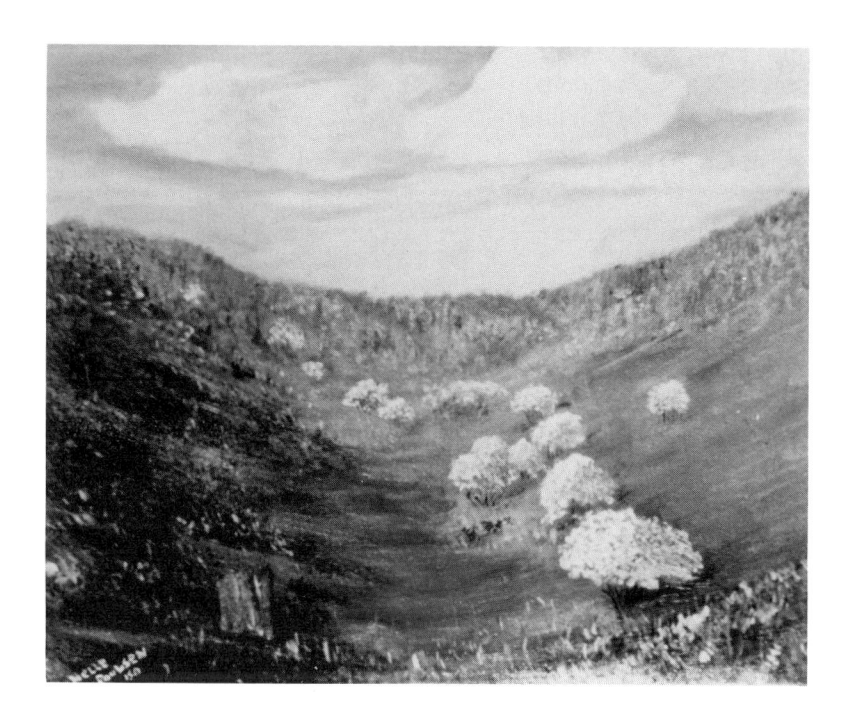

Sheridan Valley

The East have their dogwood and the South the magnolias, but in our part of the country we are fortunate enough to have the shadbush. Vast orchards of heavily laden trees with blossoms of white, peach and delicate pink that perfume the evening air with subtle fragrance.

Driving along Sheridan Valley in twilight a few evenings ago, the scores of blossom laden trees, white and still, made me wish that the people who live in drabness and squalor, could spend even a brief hour in this atmosphere of holiness which seems to be the most appropriate word for such beauty. So much loveliness to warm the heart, to gather into our remembering when days are gloomy.

Shadbush, Juneberry or Serviceberry, whatever we call them, are members of the Amelanchier family. This is not only a beautiful tree, but a very useful one. Taste the fruit in July when it turns dark purple and the juice just bubbles from its ripeness. The Indians used the dried berries as a basic ingredient in their pemmican. They also mixed it with corn meal and baked small loaves as we do muffins.

The berries are good when just stewed with added lemon juice. They can also be canned for winter use. Served hot or cold they are excellent. If you are tired of fruit pies and would like to try something different, gather the Juneberries, mix with a little flour and sugar or honey, and bake as you would a blackberry pie. The flavor is almondy and different and delicious. The servings will be a little runny, so have a spoon handy. Juneberry jam is also good. Put the fruit through a food chopper. Cook as you would any other fruit. I like to add the pulp of an orange and a lemon to give tartness.

❖

Smile

I often wonder how many of us realize how much laughter can add to our good health. A smile can even brighten a sad face. Have you ever smiled, or related a humorous story to a sick person? Watch the light come into the eyes and the smile he or she gives in response. I once heard an elderly man say "laughter is the most healthful exertion; it is one of the greatest helps to digestion with which I am acquainted, and the custom prevalent among our forefathers of exciting it at table by jesters and buffoons was founded on true medical principles." Perhaps that is why we enjoy seeing a comedian and listening to the laughter of the audience. If we consider the relief we receive from laughter, and how often it breaks the gloom brought about by illness, loneliness and grief, isn't it wise to cultivate this habit when one has the ability to relieve one's own troubles and ease the sadness of others? Many years ago I had a young male customer who came into the drug store several times a week. He had a sad, solemn look in his eyes and it seemed impossible to make him smile. I later learned that he had eye trouble and was afraid of going blind. That is when I wrote the following verses and addressed them to my solemn friend.

Prayer

Lord, if for one brief moment my sight might be restored lifting my soul from its dark abyss,

I would not seek the gold from coffers poured nor the laden board with candlelight diffused—

I would not gaze upon a woman's face, knowing the wantonness that lay beneath.

The rippling sound of water would not make me stray nor the music lure me from my desire.

Show me Lord, but one small patch of blue in a morning sky, and the white wings of a dove like praying hands spread out before the morning sun.

❖

Beware When Using Herbs

Because I have received several enquiries asking if I knew what herbs to take for various ailments, I would like to repeat advice I have given to those people who drink herb teas believing they contain the answer to all ills. They don't! In fact, unless you are very sure you can recognize your herbs and are certain of their medicinal value, a cup of tea could be the end of your life.

Many of us read of an elderly couple who had been to a health spa that recommended comfry tea for arthritis. The wife picked what she thought was comfry and prepared the tea. Within the hour she was overcome with nausea, vomiting and dizziness. What she had picked was foxglove, the source of a powerful heart drug. Yes! It cured her ailment; she died.

Some people drink senna tea, because they have been informed it is a good substitute for coffee and tea. It is not. It causes severe diarrhea, and although it is a common folk remedy for constipation, it must be treated with caution and taken in small doses.

Herbal preparations, used for more than 5000 years as medicines and tonics, are still the mainstay of folk medicines throughout the world in order to cure whatever ails them. Unfortunately, many people are unaware that herbal teas may contain any number of potent chemicals that can disrupt the normal function of both body and mind. People don't realize that preparations were once available only in pharmacies. They were used as drugs and the druggist would instruct the customer how to prepare them using correct directions and extreme caution.

Beneficial teas can be made from parsley, mint, chamomile, rose hips and many other simple plants, but don't try drinking tea made with catnip or nutmeg which a doctor recently discovered one of his friends taking. Those two drugs, along with some others, contain halucinogenic substances. *Treat all herbs with caution and be on the safe side of life.*

❖

Pests On Houseplants

Seed catalogues are here and some avid gardeners have already planted onion, cabbage and tomato seeds, hoping to be ahead of neighboring gardeners. But I have heard complaints from several people regarding pests on their houseplants. Perhaps I can offer a few remedies—some as close as your kitchen shelf. Your kitchen products are cheap, safe and effective in helping promote plant growth and protecting plants from pests, and many of them are found to be just as good as many chemicals sold in garden centers.

Buttermilk: the scourge of many ornamental plants is the mite, so tiny it would take 50 of them to cover the head of a pin. And if you have the red spider mite, do try this: Mix 1/2 cup of buttermilk, 4 cups of wheat flour and 5 gallons of water. Strain through cheesecloth and spray your plants. It will even kill the eggs.

Soap effectively destroys fungus gnats, tiny black flies that may thrive in the soil of your houseplants. Make a suds of laundry soap and pour half to one cup around the top of the pots. Any soap will do but naptha works best. One of the worst pests houseplants have to contend with are the aphids and white flies that look like dandruff. They congregate on the undersides of the leaves and suck the sap; use one teaspoonful of liquid dishwashing detergent to one gallon of water. Spray the undersides of the leaves every five days until the plant is free of these pests.

If you are a smoker or use tobacco in any form, be sure to wash your hands before you touch plants of tomato, peppers, eggplants, petunias and other members of the Solanaseae family. Tobacco-mosaic virus may be on your hands and your plants will have to be destroyed. Except for the plants belonging to this particular family, nothing is better than a tea made with a few cigarette butts and a little soapsuds.

What do I use most of the time? I put a few cloves of garlic into my blender with plenty of water and blend the bejabbers out of it. Then spray my plants. They hate the stuff and so do I. But it works!

One perfect and easy way to exterminate pests, is by putting your dog's flea collar over the plant and covering it with a plastic bag for a few hours. The toxic contents of the collar will do the trick and your dog will be most grateful.

❖

Cooking with Herbs

So! You have high blood pressure and have been advised to eliminate salt and red meat from your diet and you are wondering how on earth you are going to live without these two precious commodities.

You might help bring down the price of beef and at the same time reduce your waistline, but for the sake of gourmet enthusiasts, do the job right and add some herbs to your cooking. Without salt you will taste your food and added herbs will give another dimension to your cooking. A dash of herbs will transform the blandest, most unappetizing food into something good.

What herbs? Parsley, thyme, oregano, tarragon, sage, summer savory, chives, mint and chervil, all of which may be grown on your own window sill. If, when planting time arrives you can find a spot in your garden for these delectable greens, you have the no-meat, no-salt thing licked.

Perhaps you have decided on rice pilaf with creamed salmon for dinner. Add a teaspoonful of chopped parsley and half a teaspoonful of oregano to the onion in your sauce and the whole meal will come alive.

Quiche Lorraine, which is a cheese custard pie, makes a great meal. Leave out the bacon if you wish and just use cheese, onions and a teaspoonful each of chopped parsley and sweet basil. Macaroni and cheese will have more appeal if you add chives and a little summer savory before you bake it.

Since we shall be depending upon chicken for many meals, do remember that tarragon goes hand in hand with chicken no matter how you cook it.

If using a cream sauce make your own instead of using heavily salted soups. Do some special things with that sauce. A sprinkle of curry powder, a teaspoonful each of parsley, tarragon and oregano. Here's food fit for your best friend. If you have always tossed chicken wings into the soup pot—forget it.

Chicken wings will cease to be the cheapest part of the chicken when served in this cream sauce. If served with mashed potatoes, sprinkle with cheese and a dash of herbs and put under the broiler to brown. Who said salt was necessary for good cooking?

❖

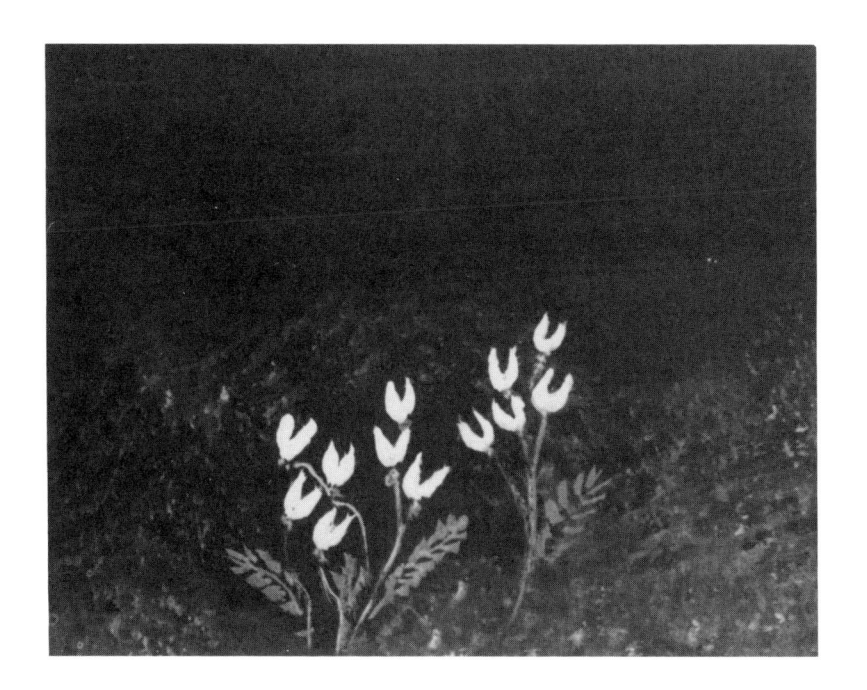

Mother Nature's Spring

Spring! So many beautiful things to see, to hear, to smell and to feel. The many shades of green, ranging from delicate chartreuse, emerald and moss, to the background beauty of pine green. Young leaves of green springing to life. Another season. Another reminder that Mother Nature is still with us. Orioles, robins and phoebes heralding the morning with inimitable song that lifts the spirit, and the sombrous creak of bull frogs to remind us that all things, even music, are laced with shadows.

Lilies of the valley, apple blossom and pin cherries wafting fragrance through the air, subduing the earthiness of decaying leaves. Wild mustard, covering the farmer's fields with a curtain of gold, while buttercups lift their yellow petals to the sun. Pastel shades of hepatica delicate loveliness that winks a greeting from the grassy banks.

Have you tasted the water from the small streams that come down from the hills? Dipped freshly gathered watercress in French dressing to delight your taste buds? Have you felt the velvet of a green bed of moss, or placed your hand on the smooth bark of a white birch? Have you held in your hand a young bird who mistook your window for sun-filled space. (I did, early this morning.) Or have you experienced the freshness of a brisk, spring wind in your hair?

❖

What Used to Be

Whatever happened to the nickel ice cream cone, the nickel cigar, candy bar and Coke. Remember when our weekly allowance was just a nickel—enough for five trips to the penny-candy counter? We could bring home a weekly wage of twenty-five dollars and live like kings—yes, even save a few dollars.

I have just spent a delightful half hour looking through a 1902 Sears catalogue. Can you believe we could buy, at that time, one hundred bars of laundry soap for $2.95? Ten pounds of Sears best coffee for $2.10; a pair of high hunting boots for $2.95? And that was high in price, for if you wished to go to a barn dance, a pair of dress shoes would set you back just $1.35!

So! You wished to buy your best girl a lacy, brocaded handkerchief, so you needed just 19 cents. Or, if father complained about feeling cold, and your sympathies were aroused, there was a suit of Australian underwear for 60 cents. And when the long underwear was packed away and summer days called for comfort, a fine French percale shirt could be purchased for 40 cents. I was interested in lace, since I recently paid 90 cents a yard. In 1902 I could have bought the same thing for 11 cents a yard. Can you imagine a 100-piece set of French Haviland china for $19.95?

What do we pay today for a good wood-burning stove? More than Sears was asking for the quality Acme in 1902. $4.29. That's right—just four dollars and twenty-nine cents.

❖

Bay Leaves

One afternoon last week, I was busy in the kitchen putting Bay leaves in strategic places, such as behind the microwave, a large cutting board, etc. I believe my friend who was watching me had an idea that I was a trifle "tetched," especially when I told her that it was to keep ants away. I don't know whether Bay doesn't like ants or whether ants don't care for the company of Bay leaves. All I know is that the two are incompatible. *Ants hate my kitchen!*

"Neither witch nor devil, nor thunder or lightning will hurt a man where a Bay tree is," said Culpepper. "They serve both for pleasure and profit, both for ornament and use, both for civil uses and for physic." All of that from the simple Bay leaf. No wonder ants run away from simple Bay leaves. In one of my old herb journals I found these words. Galen, the Greek physician said, "The leaves and bark dry and heal very much and the berries more than the leaves. It is effectual to break gallstones and open up obstructions of the liver." He also advised Bay for pestilence and other infectious diseases, rheumatic complaints, palsies, cramps and pains caused by sore traveling.

Today, we know and appreciate Bay leaves for flavoring foods. One leaf, crushed, can give a wonderful flavor to a simple dish of potatoes, onions and other vegetables and can add distinction to tomato-flavored dishes. French cooking can't be imagined without a trace of Bay, which is also one of the chief ingredients of the *Bouquet Garni*, a combination of herbs used for flavoring almost any French dish. And Bay leaves are almost as popular in all Mediterranean cooking. Add one or two leaves to chowders and soups. Use one or two Bay leaves in marinades; also to venison and other game dishes; add one or more leaves to stews, pot roasts, chicken casseroles and to the water in which ham, corned beef or tongue is cooked. Add a Bay leaf to the water in which fresh or frozen vegetables are cooked. *And don't forget the ants!*

❖

Violets

It won't be too long before the beautiful and simple violet will be blooming. Everyone welcomes this harbinger of spring, and did you know this common wildflower can make a contribution to your good health?

For many years I gathered the blossoms and crystallized them for decorating desserts, always popping every other one into my mouth. When I was very young and afternoon tea was the vogue in England, my Granny taught me to make violet sandwiches, usually for consumption by the vicar with whom she had quite a rapport. I gathered the young, tender leaves and arranged them precisely on thinly sliced homemade bread that was spread with dairy, sweet butter. Next came the blossoms laid intimately down the middle in the center of the leaves. The delicate blue of the violets gave them top honors.

The leaves and blossoms of the violet are rich in vitamins C and A. In fact, one half cup of the leaves contains as much C as three oranges. Unlike many wildflowers, the violet is not harmed by picking its blossoms, for these showy little plants produce seeds. They grow out of sheer exuberance its seems, for they multiply so rapidly the ancient Britons used to steep the blossoms in goat's milk and apply the lotion to the face to "preserve the beauty of the skin."

I came across a recipe for violet syrup a while ago. This is supposed to be a remedy for chest disorders, especially stubborn coughs.

It is easily made. Fill a jar with violet blossoms, cover with hot water and allow to stay overnight. Next day, strain, discard the blossom and add one cup of honey and the juice of a lemon. Boil the syrup for a few minutes, cool and try it. Enjoy!

❖

Knitting

I had been having severe pain in my thumbs, so I gathered knitting needles and yarn and began to knit in my few spare minutes each day. I didn't need Carpal Tunnel Syndrome or arthritic fingers, so I thought I'd try the exercise of knitting. I watched as my forefingers hurried back and forth with the rest of the fingers just naturally moving with them and two thumbs bossing the whole job. If exercise worked, this would do it. One of my friends who was a knitter once told me, "Knitting's calming effect is only one of its therapeutic benefits. It also helps overcome arthritis and builds self esteem. When you work and you are creating, you haven't got time to think of your problems. Worries just melt away." Knitting therapy isn't just for women or for arthritis. If you think any man who dabbles in needlecraft is a sissy, take a look at Rosey Grier and think again. The 300-pound, 6-foot-5-inch former defensive tackle for the Rams and New York Giants football teams does knitting and needlepoint as a hobby and lugs a bag of yarn along wherever he goes. "Don't knock it till you've tried it," he advises. John Hager, owner of a craft shop in Philadelphia has been teaching knitting for several years. He neither looks nor sounds as though he just turned fifty. He started knitting on a dare—only in his case he made it into a profession.

Dr. Herbert Benson tells us in his book *Relaxation*, a book which contains his widely acclaimed meditative instructions, that many people feel completely relaxed when knitting and that it counteracts the harmful effect of stress and can add years to your life.

I wonder who'd like a pair of mittens for Christmas?

❖

Foxglove

I've planted foxglove. I love the bell-shaped blossoms that hang down the stalks and the beautiful colors that brighten the perrenial beds in mid summer.

But, as I plant, I think of the old lady in Shropshire, England, who, 200 years ago, discovered the marvelous therapeutic value of the young leaves of this plant. How many lives have been saved by the use of digitalis, which is the active ingredient of the lovely foxglove.

The foxglove grows freely across the United States, but until recently, most of the digitalis leaves in commerce were gathered from wild plants in Oregon, Washington, New York and Europe. But because the glucosides of digitalis are fragile constituents, and in order to ensure standard potency in the end product, S. B. Penick and Co., which supplies over three quarters of the digitalis used in this country, began cultivating it on their Meadow Springs Farm in Oley, Pennsylvania.

Here the foxglove is grown as an annual from new seedlings each year, as only the first-year leaves are used. These are picked by hand in the autumn, spread on trays to dry over special ovens, then they are packed under pressure for shipment. This farm produces each year enough leaves for pharmaceutical manufacturers to make 250,000,000 tablets.

Digitalis, the wonderful drug made from the beautiful foxglove, has proven to be one of the most valuable drugs used in cardiac cases, but in recent years it has proven to be efficacious in many other illnesses.

In the late 1700's Dr. William Withering wrote: *"The Foxglove leaves, with caution given. Another proof of favouring Heaven, will happily display, the rapid pulse it can abate: and blest by him whose will is fate may give a lengthened day."*

❖

Rosemary

There's a pungent, delightful fragrance in the house today, for I have a long line of rosemary drying in a passageway. A friend, living in Florida, knowing my love for this herb, sent me a large quantity of clippings when he pruned his bushes, since it is rather difficult to grow in our climate, and it is a most welcome gift.

Whenever I smell rosemary, I am back in the kitchen of my Granny, inhaling the fragrance of roast pork or a leg of lamb well-laced with rosemary and shallots. And I recall the large pitcher of steeped rosemary leaves which Granny prepared for a woman who had lost all her hair because of a fever. The lotion was applied many times a day until enough hair had grown to brush and comb again.

Rosemary was brought to this country before 1620 by Captain John Mason, but it has been grown in European countries, particularly in France and Italy for centuries. In these countries it is used to flavor sausages and other chopped meats, and also for use in mixed pickling spices.

In England, a few chopped leaves were always added to wedding cakes, and sprigs of rosemary were a part of funeral wreaths. I make a potpourri from an old recipe my Granny used and that, too, contains rosemary. It has long been an ingredient in eau de cologne and was always used to flavor wine and ale.

For a long time it had the reputation of being a *disinfectant* and Roman physicians regarded it as being particularly effective in restoring speech after a stroke.

Hungary Water, long famous for diseases of the brain and for gout, was also made from rosemary. This was invented for Elizabeth, Queen of Hungary, and was made from rosemary steeped in spirits of wine. This special water was said to have completely cured the paralyzed limbs of the Queen.

There is an old belief that "If a maid is curious as to her future, she may obtain information by dipping a spray of rosemary in a mixture of wine, gin, rum vinegar and water in a vessel of ground glass. She is to observe this rite in the company of two other maids all under 21 years old. Having fastened the sprigs to their bosoms and taken three sips of tonic—sips are quite enough—all three rest in the same beds. The dreams that follow will be prophetic." I'll bet they were!

Well, I feel safe with my supply of rosemary, for everyone—but EVERYONE—knows no witches or evil spirits will visit a home where rosemary abounds.

❖

Healing Aloe

Last night I accidentally scalded my fingers with boiling water. I quickly applied Aloe Vera and just wrapped tissue around the fingers. In less than an hour all pain had gone and this morning the fingers look and feel as if nothing had occured to injure them. That is when I said "Thank God for Aloe Vera."

For over 3500 years, tales of "healing Aloe Vera plants" have been handed down by those who have received benefit from the juice of this plant. The Bible states that the body of Christ, when removed from the cross, was wrapped in Aloe and Myrrh and we find Aloe Vera mysteriously appearing in every phase of history with many testimonials to its great medicinal value. There are testimonials coming from the medical profession today in which they laud the value of this plant for treating burns, scalds, insect bites, mouth sores, open wounds and so many other ailments.

Some testimonials tell of oral treatment with Aloe such as stomach ulcers, constipation, colon troubles, kidney troubles, indigestion, etc. During the last thirty years, research programs with Aloe Vera have taken place in many parts of the world. Surprisingly, the U. S. S. R. has been the leader by far in this research.

Many of our plants are deservedly popular, and Aloe is one of the most deserving of them all.

Nearly every cosmetic counter carries shampoos and skin creams containing Aloe Vera. The one used for burns, etc. is just plain Aloe gel which comes in a bottle the same shape as the face lotion. Many people keep a pot of the plant growing in the kitchen. The fresh juice squeezed from a broken Aloe leaf provides instant relief for minor burns and wounds. (I have plants I would like to give away.)

❖

Parsley

I was planting parsley seed in two large pans when my grandson asked "What are you doing?" Well, I have been doing just that for many years, for parsley is a must in many foods I enjoy. I'm a bug about certain herbs and, although I have written about this versatile herb before the story bears repeating.

When we consider that 5,500 different chemicals are used in the food we eat, it is refreshing and reassuring to clip a bunch of parsley with which to add flavor to dinner, instead of monosodium glutamate and some other so-called necessaries.

Parsley enhances so many foods. Chopped parsley in scrambled eggs, cheese omelets, muffins, soups and salads and sauces. Tucked into meat stuffings. Why parsley? The ancients prized it as a medicinal. One ounce contains 22,500 units of vitamin A. This substantiates the theory of the ancients that it was an eye medicine. Carrots, which were given to flyers to overcome night blindness contained 275 units of vitamin A. How much more effective is parsley.

Parsley is also the third richest source of vitamin C. Following closely red peppers with 1,380 units per ounce, green peppers with 1,080 units, parsley has 1,050 units. Lemon juice has 360 per ounce and orange juice 270. Parsley is also the richest source of iron of all vegetables for it contains 5,763 units per ounce while spinach has but 1.2. Parsley is also rich in chlorophyll, the healing green of plants, which is, in reality, conserved sunshine.

Why do I grow parsley all winter? Because I am interested in food values. Parsley tea, with a dash of lemon and honey can almost make me *purr!*

❖

Good Readers

I took part in a conversation some time ago which interested me very much. A mother of three children was explaining why the library had been of such great help to her, and why her family patronized the library so frequently. She said that when her son, John, was a small child, she read to him every day. By the time he was ready to enter school he was a good reader and enjoyed books on many subjects. Today he is an all A student on the dean's list in college.

The second child, a girl, created problems for she too, wanted to read the books her brother found so engrossing. But mother had little time to read to her daughter. However, John read to her and someone managed to stimulate the same love of books in his sister. This would have been fine, but another "act of God" brought a boy when the other children were in their teens. Raising teens isn't exactly a "cushy" job and finding time to read to the late arrival was impossible. He started school; flunked the first grade and made no progress in the second. That was when mother decided to take over. Dismissing seemingly important things, she found time each day to read to her youngest. "It was slow going," she said, but at the end of six months, he was reading, asking for books and accompanying her to the library where he chose his own books. Today he is a good scholar—not an all A student, but good.

This conversation brought to my mind many similar instances where parents who were good readers were able to instill this love of literature in their children.

There is no better way, no easier or more interesting way to acquire knowledge than through books. Lectures by educators? Yes, they are good, but a concentrating nose-in-a-book child is closer to the subject and less likely to let the essential filter through his mind.

❖

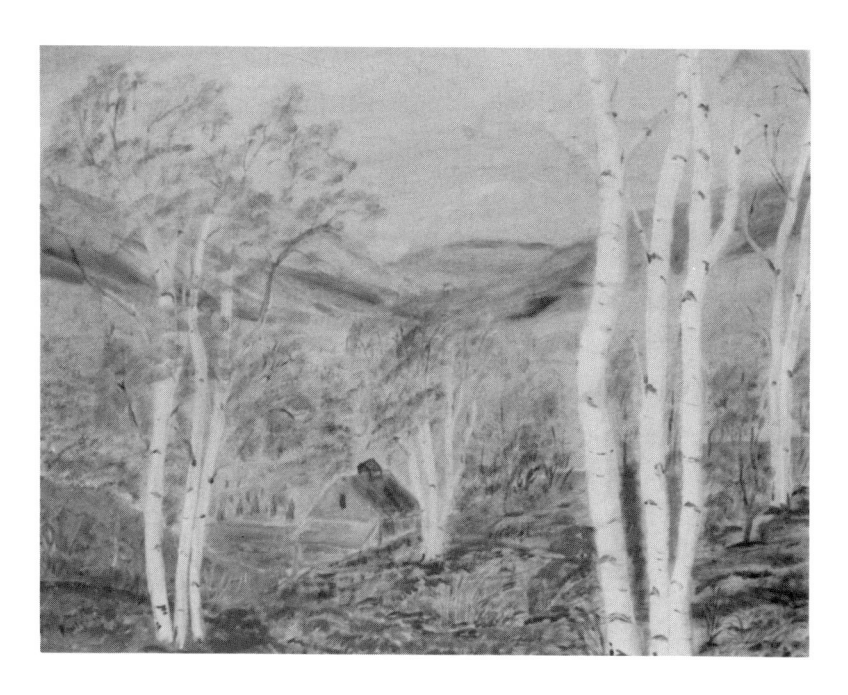

The Miracle of Life

The woods are alive with bird song. The morning sky looked as if angel wings, dipped in white paint, had brushed a pattern across the azure blue. There was a stillness in the earth that was therapy.

At my feet trilliums and violets grew profusely, and there was an abundance of flowering bushes, each one standing on tiptoe, their flower faces turned to the azure skies. Across the clearing stood a hickory tree, gaunt, and shaggy with age.

Reaching down, I gathered bright red berries of wintergreen and slowly savored their pungent flesh, remembering that wintergreen, or gaultheria, as I was taught to name it, was good for rheumatism. I wondered what, in this verdant earth, did not have some therapeutic value. The sphagnum moss at my feet, would so effectively stop bleeding as an emergency application to a wound. There is also good evidence that it contains iodine and healing acid properties. It is also quite sterile when found in a remote swamp. There's a patch of fireweed across the clearing which will soon be bearing its lovely lavender flowers.

Fireweed is rich in vitamin K which will control internal bleeding. The leaves of the trailing arbutus, now losing its fragrant blossoms, can be successfully used in urinary troubles. Yarrow, which contains the active principle insulin from which insulin derived its name, will be bringing beauty to the wood's roads very soon.

Mother Nature! Gracious, generous, forgiving. We cut down your trees, pollute your streams, desecrate the floors of your forests with litter, but the generous heart of you renews life each spring. The miracle of green, the flamboyant and fragrant blossoms. The sound of frogs, birds, and the gentle winds that stir the trees and make melody.

Life renewed! The miracle of life!

❖

Cattails

I guess I must be classified as an optimist, for I stopped to look at a bit of wetland a few days ago. I wanted to see if the cattails were showing green; of course they weren't. But this is the time of year when we think of the "wild things" and the fresh taste they give to our jaded palates after the humdrum provender of winter. I can't remember how young I was when I first went with my Granny to hunt cattails. We didn't call them cattails, though, for that would have dimmed my enthusiasm. To us, they were Lords and Ladies, but they tasted like the foods with other names such as Cossack asparagus, bull rushes, cat o' nine-tails.

One of my best taste-memories is the first spears of the cattails, lightly boiled until just tender, and served with melted butter. When the flower heads are still green, wash them in salt water, and either steam them or simmer for a short time. Try serving them with sausage links or meatballs.

If you are a dandelion fan, don't pour weedkiller on your lawn, but cut the young, tender leaves and treat them to a dose of hot dressing. Dice a rasher of bacon until crisp, pour off some of the fat and add vinegar in which you have dissolved a small amount of cornstarch and about a teaspoonful of honey. Heat the entire mixture and pour over leaf lettuce or dandelion leaves. I add a few snippets of chives. This is a salad to enjoy at the beginning of a meal, for the dressing should be quite warm.

Young, tender dandelion leaves can also be used to add character to scrambled eggs. Mix four eggs and four tablespoons of cold water with salt and pepper to taste. Add one cup of shredded dandelion leaves. Heat a little butter or bacon fat in a frying pan and add the egg mixture. When it begins to set, stir constantly, but keep them soft and creamy.

Don't forget to look for Jerusalem artichokes. They should be dug as early as possible unless you harvested them all winter as most of us do!

The miracle of greens! Enjoy them!

❖

Vitamin B1

A few days ago I had an interesting conversation with a friend about vitamin B1, so I thought I might again write about the extra things I have learned about this interesting vitamin. Many of us have reason to be thankful for the benefits received from B1. Thiamin hydrochloride, which is the chemical name of this vitamin, is a component of the germ and bran of wheat, the husk of rice, and that portion of all grains which is commercially milled away to give the grain a lighter color and finer texture. Known as the "morale vitamin" because of its relation to a healthy nervous system and its beneficial effect on mental attitude, thiamin is also linked with improving individual learning capacity. It is necessary for consistent growth in children and for the improvement in muscle tone in the stomach, the intestines and the heart. A diet rich in brewers yeast, wheat germ, blackstrap molasses and bran, will supply the body with adequate thiamin and will help prevent undue accumulation of fatty deposits in the artery wall. Thiamin is not stored in the body in any great quantity and therefore must be supplied daily. It is excreted in the urine in amounts that reflect the intake and the quantity stored.

First signs of vitamin B1 deficiency include easy fatigue, loss of appetite, irritability, and emotional instability. If the deficiency is not arrested, confusion and loss of memory appear, followed closely by gastric distress, abdominal pains and constipation. Thiamin deficiency affects the cardiovascular system as well, and indigestion, severe constipation and loss of appetite.

This vitamin has been used in the treatment of multiple sclerosis. It has improved people's dispositions by alleviating fatigue and it also improves muscle tone in the stomach and intestines. Thiamin (B1) also is given to increase energy, which is why I am now going to take my daily dose of my favorite vitamin.

❖

Sounds of Spring

The sounds of spring! The early-morning call of the phoebe, pleading and mournful. Robins proclaiming to the bird population that territory has been established, interspersing the acclaim with melodious mating music guaranteed to arouse the deepest sleeper.

Yesterday I watched a flicker as he inspected a hole made in a fence-pole by a woodpecker. He brought a female to inspect his find, but she scornfully flew away. Swallows have taken possession of the martin house and are busy carrying nest-building material. The loons send their melancholy calls across the lake and when evening arrives we'll hear eerie night sounds that split the silence of darkness. A pair of ducks have built on the shore and their noisy chatter brings aliveness to the swamp. A coyote calls from the distant hills and is not answered, but his persistence will surely bear fruit. In late afternoon, I stood quietly outside and listened to a rustle under the pines. What kind of animal can it be, I ask, and as I look closely, a pair of partridge appear, searching pine needles and dead leaves, indifferent to my presence.

It will soon be time for the shadbush to bloom with its delicate blossoms of white, palest pink and peach. There will be a symphony of honey-bee sounds, and, as if to give a final fillip to the wonderful sounds of spring, the orioles will sit atop a tree and fill the world with ecstatic sounds.

Helen Keller, blind and deaf from the age of two, gave us this advice: "I who am blind can give one hint to those who see, one admonition to those who would make full use of the gift of sight. Use your eyes as if tomorrow you would be stricken blind. And the same method can be applied to the other senses. Hear the music of voices, the song of birds, the mighty strains of an orchestra, as if you would be stricken deaf tomorrow. Touch each object you want to touch as if tomorrow your tactile sense would fail. Smell the perfume of flowers, taste with relish each morsel as if tomorrow you could never taste or smell again."

Voices

Voices! Who isn't cognizant of the effect of voices upon our sensitivity? Last week, as I left a store, the clerk said, "Have a nice day." I should have thanked him and smiled, but I felt as if I had just been sentenced to a life of loneliness. Fortunately, my next encounter was with a girl who smiled, wished me "Good morning" with joie de vivre in her voice which made the day joyful again.

There is so much power in a smile and the tone of voice we use. Even a reprimand given in the right tone, loses some of its sting and is far more effective than an abrasive voice.

How do you respond to a high, querilous voice—after your nerves have quieted down? Or that loud conversationalist who hammers out each word with the precision of a riveter, and usually embellishes the sentences with a cuss word or two. Hold your temper in obeyance. The next orator may be what I refer to as the "pussycatter," who speaks in a soft undertone laying each sentence down as if it were too hot to be touched. That is usually the "holier-than-thou" gossip who wishes to keep her spicy news from the ears of any but the privileged. Voices! What a difference they can make to the listener.

I had a friend who would look me in the eye after I had related a bit of Irishism and call me "faker" and I wanted to hug him, for his voice had no scolding.

Our voice is one of our greatest assets and when we lace its tonality with happiness and laughter, we are indeed the possessors of contentment. Henry Ward Beecher said "A man without laughter is like a wagon without springs—he is jolted disagreeably by every pebble in the road."

❖

Dandelion

As I looked over a large patch of golden dandelions a few days ago, I wondered how many people really knew the value of this plant. I do not think it is an exaggeration to say that this vitamin-filled wild plant has, over the centuries, probably saved a good many lives. But how the mighty have fallen! This herbal hero, one of the most healthful and genuinely useful plants, is now a despised lawn weed. Now, every garden supply house has several items to help exterminate these little plants which have so benefited the human race.

The finest glass of wine I ever drank was made from the golden blossoms of the dandelion; and the most interesting salad consisted of very young dandelion leaves, watercress, grated cheese and crumbled bacon. Nearly everyone has heard that dandelion leaves are edible, but the actual gathering and preparation of them seems to be an almost forgotten art. The best dandelions are never found in closely mowed lawns, but in some place where they and the grass have been allowed to grow freely.

The dandelion plant is a great supplier of vitamins A and C. It is also an excellent source of Calcium and Potassium. Isn't it ironic that we spend so much on herbicides to kill this delectable source of nutrients? Dandelions are the richest and most palatable of all vegetables and it is still the favorite green of thousands of people who eat it every spring. It is held in high esteem in Britain, and in France it is sold in the markets.

The dandelion's medicinal uses are chiefly for stimulating the kidneys and bladder and as a general tonic, so don't push aside this delightful herb as being useless except to annoy lawn growers who consider a good lawn without weeds a mark of prestige.

I cook the young leaves as you would spinach. Use very little water and drain well. I add a few chopped chives and a little butter. I wish I had a little dandelion wine to accompany this vegetable to my tummy!

❖

Fiddleheads

If you were in New England right now and dining in a fine restaurant, you would undoubtedly find on the menu, fiddleheads. And, of course, you would order these delectable greens for there is nothing to surpass their elegant flavor. We, too, have fiddleheads and they are to be harvested along the lovely streams of Michigan—especially *our* part of Michigan.

Not all ferns, which unfold in a shape resembling fiddleheads are edible, but the ostrich fern, which are abundant in this part of the country, are considered to be the finest.

The ostrich fern fiddleheads are ready for harvesting when their stems are from two to five inches long and their thick crosiers are still unfurled. Snap them off about two inches above the roots. Fiddleheads are reminiscent of asparagus and morels. They have a pleasing taste that is readily accepted by anyone who loves vegetables.

They need to be washed in lots of cool water to remove the brown scales that cover the fiddleheads as they rise from the earth. Some of them can be rubbed off or even blown off, but there are stubborn scales that must be removed by washing and by hand rubbing. However much work you put into the preparation it is indeed worth while.

A great luncheon dish may be prepared with hot buttered toast covered with crisp fried bacon and covered again with cooked fiddleheads. Fiddleheads in a quiche, in a salad, in souffles, soups, and as a vegetable are indeed a delight.

❖

Sage

I managed to walk into my garden this morning and greet the first herbs of spring. Tarragon, oregano, thyme, chervil, lemon balm and the many mints. There was a bush of sage I planted last year, its dew-covered leaves glistening in the sun, and I thought of the many uses to which we put this beautiful herb.

It is one of the strong herbs and so should be used with discretion. However, many folks think it is used only for dressings for poultry or for flavoring sauces. The finest chefs use this herb in small quantities with many different meats—pork, veal and even with some cuts of beef. Sage vinegar is excellent for use in mayonnaise and salad dressings.

The ancient herbalists valued sage for many other reasons. They used it for tuberculosis, believing it was an enemy of all germs. An infusion of this herb is used for washing wounds. It dissolves uric acid, thus it helps cure rheumatism. As a gargle for sore throat it is most effective. Should you be a brunette, a sage rinse will help keep your tresses dark.

The word sage means wise. Evidently we stole it from the French and this makes sense when we are told that its use is said to improve and strengthen the memory and to clear the brain.

There is a quotation which states, "Why should man die when he has sage in his garden." In fact, this line is on many old English tombstones. The Chinese are great users of sage and seem to prefer sage tea to their own.

King Solomon is said to have praised the use of sage along with rosemary and rue. Besides being a singer of songs, the good king was also a great horticulturist and knew more about plants than any other man in his time. He speaks of birds, herbs, flowers and trees. With 600 wives, he probably found it prudent to retire to the woods on many occasions. It is interesting to know that the ancients used the same herbs we use today. Guess I'll begin using sage in my salad. Perhaps it will help me to remember what happened to the month of May.

Honey

I have just finished my breakfast of oatmeal, sliced banana and a tablespoon of honey. In these days when we are constantly being warned about the additives in our food, it's a relief to know there is at least one pure food, honey! Here is a food that remains stable. Apparently bees have more sense than humans. Here are some facts about honey. Records show that it was used in cave-dwelling days, and for ages, the one food of pure sweetening available, was the product of the bee. Honey contains the minerals and vitamins so necessary to good health, and they are all derived from the soil in which plants grow, are passed from the plants to the nectar of the flowers to be used by the bee.

Honey is especially beneficial to people who suffer from gastrointestinal distress, for, unlike cane sugar and starches which have to be converted into simple sugars, all of which add extra work for the stomach, honey has been processed by the bees.

Many physicians recommend honey because it is non-irritating to the lining of the digestive tract. It quickly supplies energy to the body so is especially beneficial to the athlete. It is, of all sweeteners, handled best by the kidneys. It also has a sedative action, so two teaspoonfuls of honey in a glass of warm water at bedtime will deprive you of all thoughts of a sleeping pill. If you have a cough, try equal parts of honey, glycerin and lemon juice, and if you are not a teetotaler, substitute the glycerin with something much more effective, whiskey.

For arthritic pains, try an eight ounce glass of water to which has been added two teaspoons of honey and one of cider vinegar. A refreshing therapeutic. Because of the high content of vitamin C in honey, it is wonderful in controlling leg cramps. On a diet? Cheer up. A teaspoonful at the end of a light meal will give a feeling of fullness.

Honey! I wonder why we call a person we love by that five letter word?

❖

A Snowy Owl

At first I thought it was a piece of lingerie which had been whipped by the wind and fastened its whiteness around the top of the fence post. Then as I looked closer, a pair of extraordinary yellow eyes fixed themselves upon me. There was a slight movement and I noticed a few transverse bars of slate brown across what I suddenly realized was a snowy owl.

Strangely enough, my husband and I saw a snowy owl in exactly this spot about seven years ago, but I had never been so close to one. It was so still, so picturesque. It sat like a white specter atop the post and I sat equally silent, for I wanted to see what this strange bird would do.

Its gaze never seemed to falter from my face and I wondered what thoughts—if birds can think—were racing around in that snowy poll. I remembered reading that this owl was most useful to farmers, destroying mice, rats and other rodents. It is also very fond of fish and is able to catch them alive. Its flight is so swift it is able to capture a grouse when in flight, but what, I wondered, could it find to eat in this territory at this time of year.

A clear, vibrant croaking noise cut through the stillness and I quickly glanced around to see what was approaching, not realizing the sound came from the snowy bundle in front of me. Then those eyes came alive and swift as an arrow the snowy owl sailed into the air. I opened the car door and stood watching as the bird dropped into the corn field of the farm. What could he possibly find there and how had he been able to observe anything from such a distance?

There was a light snow falling and the world was very still. It was then I heard the cry of pain and I knew that snowy owl had caught a small animal and so found his lunch.

❖

Roses

I cannot leave the story of the rose without adding a few of the many uses to which this flower adds elegance.

The petals of all the heavily scented varieties are the heart and soul of many sachets, perfumes, flower teas and potpourris. The culinary uses of the rose petals are probably the most exotic of all the herbs, and their culinary history dates back into ancient times.

The Persians made a heady wine from the petals of roses, and during the 12th Century in England a rose-petal liqueur was a rare and exotic delicacy. Today, in England the petals of roses are candied, or they are made into jam as they are in India.

The French attar of roses is perhaps the most fragrant of all the attars of roses. The skill of the French in preparing the oil of roses and rose water is world renowned and has made France a leader in the preparation of perfumes. However, oil of roses and rosewater also provide extremely subtle and delicate flavoring in fancy cakes and cookies. The French have also developed a rose petal vinegar which is an aged cider vinegar seasoned with herbs and rose petals.

Homemakers today who are eager to add an imaginative touch and a subtle taste to various herb teas will discover that by blending a few heavily scented rose petals with them an extraordinarily flavor and aroma are given to the teas. A fruit cup or a fruit salad, or a jelly flavored with the petals can be one of the most delightful taste experiences.

Here is an old-time recipe for rose jelly. Do try it: 2 $1/2$ cups canned apple juice; 1 quart fresh rose petals, tightly packed; 3 $1/2$ cups sugar; $1/2$ bottle Certo; red food coloring.

Heat juice to boiling point but do not boil. Pour hot juice over well washed petals. Boil 30 minutes then drain off juice into another pan. Add sugar, stir, and add two drops of coloring. Bring to boil and add Certo. Boil one minute more; pour into sterile glasses.

Yogurt

"How can anyone eat that stuff?" Those were words of a woman speaking to her companion as they watched me pick up two cartons of yogurt in the grocery store.

The staple of peasants and the delicacy of kings, and so delicious you almost forget how good it is. Can you believe those words were spoken of yogurt? The people who say they hate yogurt have often never tried it. But today, yogurt is a food that is given credit for curing such things as high cholesterol levels, arthritis, constipation, diarrhea, gallstones, halitosis, and kidney disorders. Yogurt contains the B-complex vitamins, and has a higher percentage of A and D than does the milk it is made from. It is also high in protein.

The Old Testament tells of Abraham waxing strong on goat's milk yogurt, and it was probably responsible for Sarah's long reproductive cycle. Solomon's wisdom is surely somewhere responsible to his consumption of yogurt. And ask the Bulgarians why Methuselah lived to such a ripe old age. Earlier than the third century, Persians were making yogurt from the milk of goats, sheep, camels and water buffalo. Genghis Khan, it is reported, devoured yogurt by the crockful, fed it to his armies, and used it to preserve meat. There is evidence to support the notion that the Mongol hordes poured fresh milk into their saddle bags and let the heat of their steeds' bodies work the milk into yogurt.

Many years ago, I had a telephone call from a doctor who ordered yogurt for a woman who was one of my customers suffering from vaginal yeast infection. I found a recipe for yogurt which my customer made and from which she certainly benefited. Yesterday, in a health letter, I read that yogurt was being used for burns, cold sores, facial skin care and vaginal infections.

I guess I'll have a dish of yogurt at lunch time, and I'll embellish it with a spoonful of creme de menthe.

❖

Vitamin C

I have just taken my daily dose of vitamin C. For many years I have been interested in vitamin C and its therapeutic value, and perhaps because I am a pharmacist, I am always seeking knowledge relating to my profession. I read everything I can find that gives authentic information about the drugs that have been such an integral part of my life.

Long before vitamin C was made synthetically, even before it was known as a vitamin, I asked my friends to eat lots of rose hips, parsley, watercress, etc. because my beautiful, witching Granny taught me the value of these things. Growing pains, charlie horses, and what we today call bursitis were all wished away with large doses of vitamin C bearing herbs.

Recently, I read this bit of heartening news in an English paper: "A study at St. Paul's Hospital in London, conducted by two famous doctors, appears to have proven that vitamin C is the best, and perhaps the only valid, preventative of bladder cancer. The study is based on the discovery that the urine of cigarette smokers is luminescent and excites a positive reaction in a geiger counter. It appears that bladder cancer is confined almost exclusively to cigarette smokers and the researchers are investigating the hypothesis that malignant changes in the bladder are caused by some as yet unknown radioactive substances in tobacco. Smokers whose daily diet includes substantial amounts of vitamin C, however, do not have the same luminescence and radioactivity in their urine and a direct connection has been established."

That information is certainly worth consideration. Think of it next time you reach for a cigarette.

Don't forget that all green vegetables contain vitamin C. So do strawberries, apples, citrus fruits of all kinds and lots of parsley should be a daily part of your diet. *Happy eating!*

❖

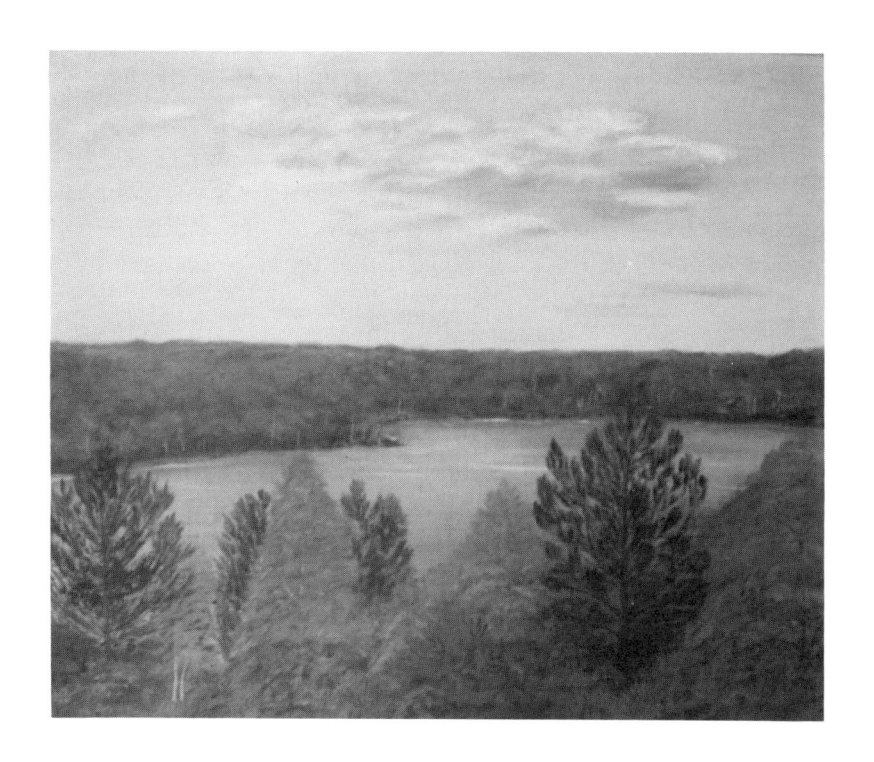

The Day Is Done

Last evening I sat on the porch, 180 feet above the lake. The day had been hot and humid, but an evening breeze came in from the west, soft as a caress—and as welcome. The curtains of twilight veiled the surrounding woods, but slowly dissipated to reveal the dark, velvety heavens of night. Behind me, the moon rose slowly above the horizon casting fantastic shadows from the trees and putting whimsical patterns on the water of the lake. A shooting star reminded me that there are places above this earth.

There was a stillness that wrapped itself around my body, like a comforting cloak on a bitter cold day, and I think of the city, moody and provocative as a mistress, restless as the elements, where loves and hates run rife and only the strong survive the fray. As darkness waited for the moon to appear there was a hushed silence over everything. The world slowly came alive with beauty and shadows changed their course. What a world! Magnificent solitude of our north woods! There were soft rustlings in the underbrush as small animals hastened to their resting places, and two deer walked slowly down the path to the lake, wary of the woman who sat on the porch. A tree toad said "goodnight" with startling clarity and a loon flapped its wings in the water of the lake. Night sounds! Perhaps the only sounds we really enjoy. The weird call of a coyote and the cry of a startled bird. The far away drone of a truck carrying food to the city, a reminder that even this oasis of peace would end.

As I walk into the house, I think of the words of Longfellow: *"The day is done, and the darkness falls from the wings of night, as a feather is wafted downward from an eagle in his flight."*

❖

Plants' Emotions

In case you might, at times, think you are going dotty if you should happen to be caught talking to your houseplants—never fear! You are perfectly normal and perhaps smarter than those who think you are off your rocker. I have been reading a book given to me by my daughter, who is also one of those people who converse with nature. This story, entitled *The Secret Life of Plants*, very convincingly tells of the astonishing reaction of plants to various stimuli.

Scientist Marcel Vogel began some remarkable experiments with plants. When he asked his seminar students "Do plants have emotions?" he was met with derision, but also curiosity. He had obtained an instrument called a "psychanalyser" which would pick up and amplify reactions from plants. In one of Vogel's experiments he asked a friend who had tried using chemicals to find out how plants reacted. Since she had no success, she was urged to experiment with leaves. Back in her garden, Vivian Wiley picked two leaves from a saxifrage plant, one of which she put on her bedside table, the other in the living room. "Each day, when I get up," she told Vogel, "I look at the leaf by my bed and will it to live, but I pay no attention to the other." A month later, she called Vogel and asked him to bring a camera to photograph the leaves. The leaf by the bedside was radiantly vital and green, but the one that had been neglected was brown and decaying. Unbelievable? You bet!

Vogel also discovered that some of the philodendrons he worked with had their own personality and individuality. His plants seem to go through phases of activity and inactivity. In lecturing to a group of college students, Vogel made this statement, "It is a fact, man can and does communicate with plant life. Plants are living objects, sensitive, rooted in space. They may be blind, deaf and dumb in the human sense, but there is no doubt in my mind that they are very intelligent." Some humans are temperamental and so are animals, but plants really flummox me.

Mint

Having just finished drying and grinding four bushels of parsley, along with various amounts of thyme, oregano, tarragon, lemon balm etc. I was happy to get to the fragrant, refreshing orange mint, and I wondered who first discovered this delightful herb.

The story I like is about Pluto, the god of the underworld, who, on one of his trips from home was quite taken by the beauty of the daughter of Cocytus, a nymph called Mentha. Now Pluto had a wife, Prosperine, who had little affection for her dark and surly lord who had captured her by trickery, but she still was upset by his transgression. Prosperine changed the hapless damsel into a herb, one that would grow profusely wherever men might walk, one that would be trampled underfoot.

There is a mention of mint in the New Testament, Matthew 23, "Woe unto you scribes and Pharisees, hypocrites! For ye pay tithe of mint and anise and cummin, and have omitted the weightier matters of judgement, mercy and faith."

The medicinal uses of mint are many, Rose leaves and mint, combined and heated, made a sort of poultice for the aching medieval head. Mint was also recommended for the soothing of wasp and bee stings. Mint was trodden upon by kings on their way to the throne.

And, of course, mint has made an enduring place for itself in the kitchen. Apples will soon be ripe and here is a recipe you might enjoy.

Minted Apples

In a saucepan combine 3 cups water, 1 $1/2$ cups sugar, and $3/4$ cup chopped, fresh mint. Cook the mixture for five minutes. Peel, core and quarter 6 large green apples. Drop in syrup and poach until tender.

❖

Six Senses

We have five senses, although some claim to have six. I wonder if we ever use those senses to their full capacity. Do we really see the plumage on a bird, or look into the heart of a flower. Have we ever closely observed the artistry of a spider's web or marveled at the exquisite beauty of a snowflake?

We can smell the pungency of hot vinegar, but how about bread, fresh from the oven, new mown hay, the earth after a summer shower, lilacs in bloom or the smell of home after a long absence?

Do we really taste things? Food, for instance. We chew it briefly, then down the hatch it goes. But let the delicate taste buds take over. Roll a wild strawberry or raspberry over your tongue. Let a crust of fresh bread spread with good butter linger in your mouth. The first fresh orange juice of morning, vegetables from the garden, pungent watercress from a stream; what's your hurry?

What do we listen to? Raucous music from the rock and rollers over TV and radio, or the melodious song of birds, mating call of frogs, the singing sound of insects, and the soul-satisfying symphonies of the great creators. Listen! Listen for those who call out for help, to the young, the troubled, the bewildered. Let your ears remind you that, at times, you too, needed a listener.

Have you ever touched the bark of a silver birch or stroked the feathers of a crippled bird. Have you felt the richness of velvet pile or the luxury of satin and cherished its texture? Have you ever felt the richness of bread dough melting into elasticity under the pressure of your fingers or touched the skin of a baby delicate as a flower petal?

Oh well, there's another sense. It's called intuition. I have a feeling that the intuition of some readers will label this whole page *nonsense*.

❖

Open Books, Open Doors

There are many ways of trying to tolerate the excessive heat of summer. Cool showers—which are far less effective then warm showers; a dip in the lake or membership in a nudist camp. Personally I find that a quiet spot and a good book is a real panacea.

You open doors when you open books—doors that swing wide to unlimited horizons of knowledge, wisdom and inspiration that will enlarge the dimensions of your life. Vituperative words won't lessen the heat. Cold beer won't prevent dehydration, so why not look around for a peaceful corner and make up your mind to adjust to what God wishes to send us.

Through books you can encompass in your imagination the full sweep of world history. You can watch the rise and fall of civilizations, the ebb and flow of mighty battles and the changing patterns of life through the ages. Two weeks ago I was reading a delightful book that set my memory tingling, for the locale of the novel was the small village where I lived as a child. It was also the home of a rich aristocratic family who had a secret—a secret I have wondered about many times. Now I know the secret for it was beautifully written into the romantic heart of the book I was reading. I remembered something I read a long time ago; "Through books you can start today where the great thinkers of yesterday left off, because books have immortalized man's knowledge. Thinkers, dead a thousand years, are as alive in their books today as when they walked the earth."

It isn't necessary to just read modern novels. Look in the non-fiction department of your local library. Learn about the peoples of other countries; of the beauty of Alaska and the elegance of Parisian society. Read the biographies of our own great artists, poets, writers and the men and women who have given so much of their lives for our country. With only fifteen minutes a day you can read twenty books a year. Find a quiet corner—and a good book.

Did you say the temperature was in the 90s. I never noticed!

❖

She's a Lady

"She's a lady. She's educated." That was a remark made by my Granny when I first saw the beautiful daughter of Lord Dartmouth. If an education would make me as beautiful as Lady Joan, then education was for me. For many years I walked three miles a day to school, but that was my exercise period, for in those days we were not lucky enough to have a fine gym, basketball, baseball or a marching band, and exercise was important for young limbs. We sat at our desks from 9 a.m. until 4:30 p.m. with a short period for lunch. No coffee breaks or rest periods between classes. Our concentration was upon reading, writing, arithmetic, history, geography, drawing and of course, Mr. William Shakespeare! All through those years was that determination to be educated—to be a lady! Though what the alternative to being a lady really was baffled me until I was sure I wasn't going to be a gentleman.

I was appalled a few weeks ago to learn that 53 percent of the citizens of our country were illiterate. With all the advantages and the many privileges available to everyone in our schools, how could this happen? I learned of a young lady who could take apart and put together an entire automobile, but alas, when the time came and she wished to apply for a position being advertised, she was unable to write a resume. A woman whom I greatly admire is the best cook and baker I have ever known. A while ago she wished to apply for a position as head cook in a fine hotel. But how to write an application, and what to say when she couldn't even spell.

We have schools, good schools where anyone can receive a good education. Let us do everything we can to maintain those schools and give an education with the advantages children of my early years could never hope for.

"Life has loveliness to sell, beautiful and splendid things." Shouldn't we gather that loveliness by giving all we can give to our schools?

❖

Vanilla

I just poured a small amount of vanilla from a pint bottle a friend brought to me from Mexico. I love the fragrance and thought of the many uses to which this bean is put. Vanilla belongs to the orchid family as everyone knows, but does everybody know where the finest vanilla grows? The honors go to Mexico, which competes with Madagascar, Java and Tahiti, and many other orchidaceous countries. The perfumer is heavily indebted to the vanilla.

The vanilla beans are harvested when they are still unripe but just at the point when they start to turn yellow at the end, which takes about seven months. Strangely enough, when they are picked they are odorless; it is the curing process which brings out the vanilla fragrance. There are a number of variations in this process, depending on the locale, but the following is a typical procedure.

The beans are first immersed in water at 63 degrees centigrade for several minutes, then they go into wool lined barrels. All muffled up in their wooly cocoon, the beans sweat it out for 24 hours. As if that weren't enough, they are spread out on trays covered with cloths which are exposed to the sun for a period of six hours a day for six or seven days. Now they cool off slowly in the welcome shade of large drying sheds where they are inspected every day for four to six weeks, and all the time they are getting harder and darker, and much more wrinkled. Next comes a coating of castor or olive oil to preserve them, and the final step in the curing cycle is grading, tying the beans into bundles, and packing them into parchment lined tins. From these muchly coddled vanilla beans, white crystaline needles called vanillin, can be derived. The first vanillin ever made cost 800 dollars. Today it can be bought for very little money.

Vanilla! When you make a batch of cookies, sniff gently on the flavoring, remembering what those poor beans have to endure just to give you pleasure.

❖

Work and Play

"A master in the art of living knows no sharp distinction between his work and his play, his labor and his leisure, his mind and his body, his education and his recreation. He hardly knows which is which, he simply pursues his vision of excellence through whatever he is doing and leaves others to determine whether he is working or playing. To himself he always seems to be doing both." The author of these words is unknown, but whenever anyone tells me they are bored and just "fed up" with work, these words come to mind.

I wish that those who despise work would become acquainted with the essays of Kahil Gibran in his book, *The Prophet*. Here are a few excerpts:

"You work that you may keep pace with the earth and the soul of the earth. For to be idle is to become a stranger unto the seasons, and to step out of life's procession, that marches in majesty and proud submission toward the infinite.

"When you work you are a flute through whose heart the whispering of the hours turns to music. Which of you would be a reed, dumb and silent, when all else sings together in unison?

"And to love life through labor is to be intimate with life's inmost secret. And when you work with love you bind yourself, and to one another, and to God. Work is love made visible. If you cannot work with love but only with distaste, it is better that you should leave your work and sit at the gate of the temple and take arms of those who work with joy. For if you make bread with indifference, you bake a bitter bread that feeds but half of man's hunger. And if you sing though as angels and love not the singing, you muffle man's ears to the voices of the day and the night."

I have benefited from reading these verses during my life. So! I guess I'll get back to work!

❖

Oregano

I was outside looking over my garden this morning. It is surrounded by the beautiful orchid blossoms of Oregano—flowers that will last for many weeks in water but will also dry beautifully for winter bouquets. I was a little annoyed by the way in which this herb has taken over until the day I looked at the price of a small jar of Oregano in the supermarket. Now I talk sweet nothings to it in a language they seem to understand! The word *Origabum* comes from the Greeks and translates into "joy of the mountains." Culinary and domestic uses for oregano have abounded throughout the centuries.

The Greeks sowed it on graves, and if the plants flourished, the dead were said to have found peace in afterlife, English housewives polished their furniture with its oils, and the leaves of the plant were strewn on the floors as a deodorizer. The leaves were also used to keep away moths and were placed in cupboards and drawers, or put into small sachets and liberally distributed.

Oregano was also used to flavor ale and beer before hops were used for brewing. How well I remember oregano tea which was supposed to fend off colds. Many herbalists hold this herb to be used for nervous stomachs, intestinal troubles, liver ailments, insomnia, headaches and rheumatism. Not bad for a sweet smelling herb! Oregano's popularity increased after World War II. Before this time, American cookbooks simply referred to it as "wild marjoram," but soldiers returned home from Italy with a great love for Italian pizza, and oregano is used extensively in the sauce used in pizzas. As the popularity of pizza spread throughout the United States so did the use of oregano. In cooking, dried oregano may be used in place of the fresh variety, but just half of the dried is enough for it will overpower other flavors if not carefully measured.

This herb goes well with vegetables, meats, chicken, spaghetti, shrimp, baked fish, and yes—even bread. Just try it!

❖

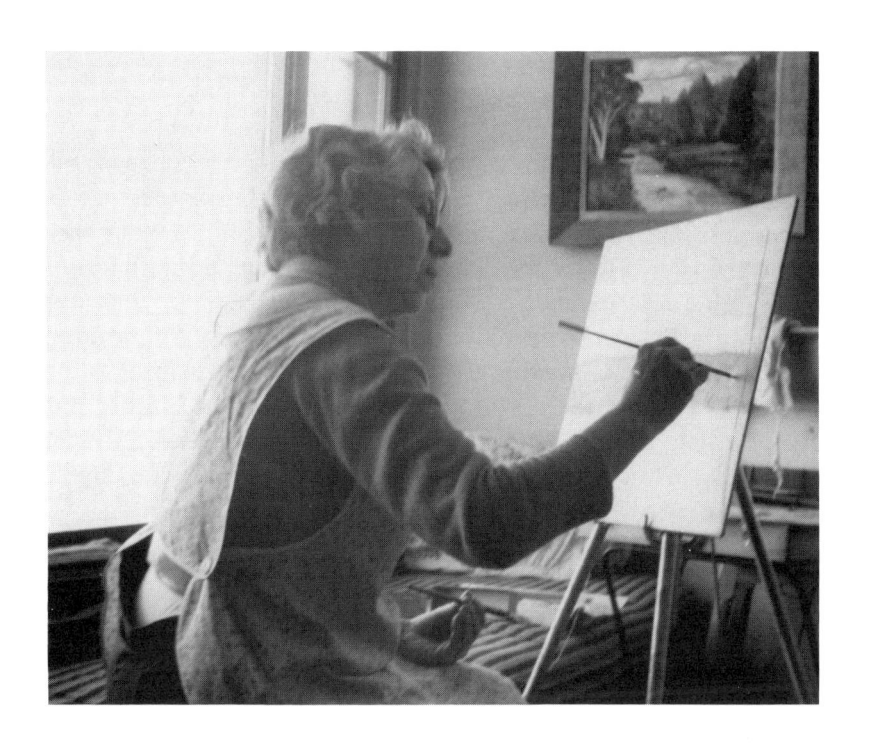

I Like to Paint!

I have often been asked why I am so interested in painting and when did I first paint a picture. I think it was when I began to realize all my thoughts and activities were tied up in just one subject, pharmacy, and all that went with it day after day, year after year. I became ill, but I found time to think and my thinking led me to consider a hobby with which to diversify my thinking. I began to paint.

Many remedies are suggested for the avoidance of worry and mental strain by persons who, over prolonged periods, have to bear exceptional responsibilities and discharge duties on a very large scale. Some advise exercise, and others repose. Some counsel travel, and others retreat. Some praise solitude, and others gaiety. No doubt all these play their part according to the individual temperament. The cultivation of a hobby and new forms of interest is therefore a policy of first importance, but it's not a business that can be undertaken in a day or swiftly improvised. I bless the day when painting came to my rescue—

when I could look at the sky and see the beauty in a cloud; the hope in the color of spring greens and the vital brilliance of fall. To sit and paint a snow picture is, to me a special time of peace and if the world looks too tranquil, it can be roused with a running brook or a flying bird.

Painting is complete as a distraction. I know of nothing which, without exhausting the body, more entirely absorbs the mind. To be able to reproduce the colors Mother Nature has put on earth. To mix blue and yellow and make green and soften that to meet all shades—doesn't that give one a feeling of creativity? Anyway—I like to paint!

❖

Bread

Bread! One item of food that belongs in every country. I once heard the expression, "There are parts of the world where people bake loaves beautiful as the face of Christ and pray in gratitude for their bounty." The Rumanians used to say, "The bread of my land though to others is hard and bitter, to me is sweet." The Slavs used to say, "Without bread even a palace is sad, but with bread a pine tree is paradise." To the Spaniards, "All sorrows are less with bread." To the Danish people, "Bread is better than the song of birds."

For more than forty years I baked my own bread, and as I kneaded the dough, these sayings of the people of various countries came into my head. There is something almost sensual about the kneading of dough—molding, pressing, forming, the feel of elasticity under the heel of the hand. One thinks of life being patterned and what wonderful things we can make of it if we only try.

Bread! The staff of life. The one thing that might maintain life when all else is denied.

The Puritans admitted that "Brown bread and the gospel is good fare." And who could ask for more. "A book of verses underneath the bough, a jug of wine, a loaf of bread and thou."

Bread has made history too. Bread riots unseated emperors in ancient Rome. The French revolutionists of 1789 cried for bread and received the unthinking reply, "Let them eat cake."

In all ages governments, in times of stress, have hesitated before taking the final, desperate step of rationing bread.

Well, guess I'll cut a slice of homemade bread for my lunch. "Give us this day our daily bread."

❖

Small Things in Life

As I grow older I seem to ask myself many questions which I ignored when I was younger. Why do we wait to do something big. What is wrong with the small things in life, and why do we ignore them as being inconsequential?

A smile, a handshake, an affectionate hug or a kiss. Just a moment of time, but something which can warm the heart, and bring a moment of happiness to the recipient. Is it necessary to write a long letter with never a word of love or affection until the last sentence.

A dog wags his tail, a cat tucks in all its loose ends and quietly purrs as it looks at you. A baby smiles and your heart sings. Such small things. Does your heart feel lighter when you hear an old song or a simple hymn, or do you wish for a great symphony when an old refrain which was almost forgotten comes over the radio to stir old memories.

The most beautiful flowers I ever received were not the roses or gardenias which were the gifts of beaus. What filled me with happiness I have never forgotten, was a bouquet of wild violets my little daughter gathered from the near-by woods and presented to me on a Mother's Day, long long ago.

We give of ourselves when we give gifts of the heart, love, kindness, sympathy and understanding.

Have you ever watched the faces of an elderly man or woman as they read an unexpected letter from an old friend? Beautiful isn't it?

I believe it was Emerson who said "Rings and jewels are not gifts, but apologies for gifts. The only true gift is a portion of thyself."

❖

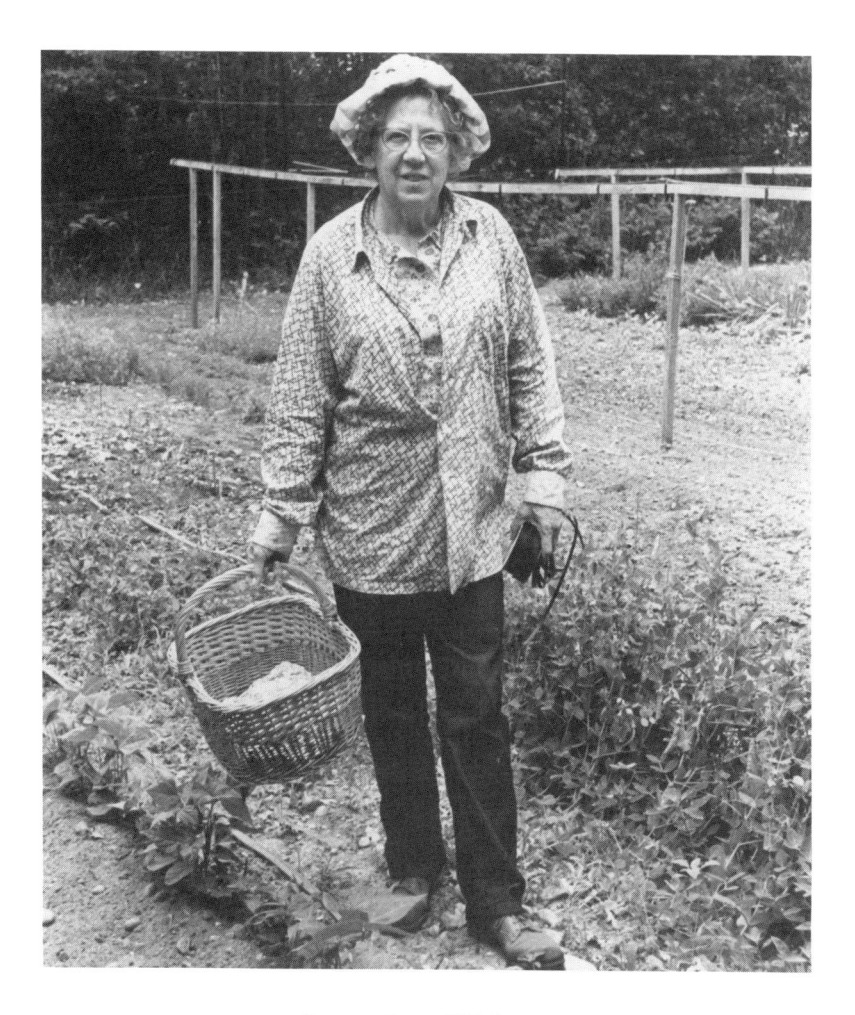

Growing Things

Gardening? What's wrong with a few aches and pains? Growing things, flowers and vegetables, is a satisfying pastime—perhaps you'll allow me to name it a profitable hobby, for have you given thought to the price you pay for not-so-fresh veggies from the store?

There's joy in handling live plants and when you can label them "life giving food" and happiness in the production of such produce. Yes! I've grunted and groaned with pain in my legs as I hoed weeds down twenty five rows of carrots, corn, beets, etc., but 89-year-old legs are privileged to complain. However, there is always a remedy.

My remedy came when a friend made me ten raised beds about four feet square. Last year I had the best beds of vegetables and herbs that I ever had from the leg-aching twenty five foot rows. Two movements! and the raised bed is weed free. How? I kneel on a soft pad, and with a small tool send the weeds to the compost heap. I move once! Of course no one realized that from such a position I can be comfortable on my knees, say my prayers, and dig up a weed at the same time. How do I find the time? I take the receiver off the telephone, inform my invalid husband I'll be in the garden just fifteen minutes, check my watch, pick up the trowel and kneel.

The complaining bird on the fence near her nest is ignored. So is the cat who tries to assure me that her method of digging is best, and I'm thankful mosquitoes seldom bite folk who take vitamin B 1. Gardening is therapy. Home grown vegetables are healthful. What more can we ask for?

——— ❖ ———

There Is Always Music

Music has always been an integral part of life from the very beginning of time. There must have been birds in the Garden of Eden. There's a thread of music running through almost every book in the Bible. What would life be like without music?

We sing when we are happy, yes, even when we are sad, although the melody may be dirge-like. Music is a safety valve, whether it be an old hymn that recalls childhood memories, the melody of a dance that ended sadly in the termination of a first love affair, ballads sung huskily by a grandparent, or a lullaby with all the nuances of love. It's music!

People protesting their enslavement sang their poignant, pensive cadences. The Israelites gave music to their beseechings. Our young radicals today are not doing anything with their strident rock and roll that generations before them haven't done. Some of the greatest music ever written was composed by men and women beset by pain, grief and sorrow, who felt the need to express themselves.

Why did I suddenly think of music as being so important to life? Because the words of the Persian poet Sadi came to mind: "If of thy mortal goods thou are bereft, and from thy slender store two loaves alone to thee are left: sell one, and with the dole, buy hyacinths to feed thy soul."

Perhaps we all need "hyacinths." Need to listen and hear the keening wind in the pine trees, the nuances of a great symphony, or the brilliance of the song of a vesper sparrow at eventide. To attune our ears to the sound of a waterfall, a woods brook, or the ponderous roll of the tide along a coastal shore... nature's music!

— ❖ —

Night Rain

Night rain! What is more fascinating? What so comforting and satisfying? I love it. A hot summer day with trees and plants begging for surcease. Night falls and stars stud the sky and heat fills every pore. Then darkness spreads its ebony across the earth and through the stillness one hears the soft patter of raindrops. The thirsty earth opens its pores and drinks the ectasy of moisture, and the heart of the listener sings, for it's a melody of relief and thirst-quenching happiness.

I think it was Ure who wrote these words "How singular, and yet how simple, the philosophy of rain. Who but the Omniscient One could have devised such an admirable arrangement for watering the earth. Sometimes there's a night of pain—physical and offtimes mental, when one wishes for the hours to speed and bring daylight. And suddenly like fairy footsteps comes the patter of small raindrops on dried leaves. Life returns. The will to keep living, the knowledge that life keeps going on—so why not us?"

To walk in the rain with face uplifted, feeling the softness of rain water—that's sheer joy. Ask the flowers, the leaves, the insects. Maybe even the birds could tell you why they sing for rain.

Very soon, the first soft snow will be falling—yes, it fell on the 23rd day of last September—lending pristine beauty to the world and spreading a blanket of protection over the resting vegetation, until spring with her magic touch awakens the world once again.

Garlic with Hollyhocks

This morning I planted garlic cloves around the hollyhocks. I imagined the rose colored blossom saying to the white one, "what on earth is she doing?" but I can't humiliate them by telling them they are harboring aphids and that garlic and aphids are incompatible.

Planting various herbs between vegetables and flowers will help keep them pest free. For instance, marigolds planted in pest harboring soil will give off a substance from its roots which kills nematodes in the soil. Sage and thyme will also drive away many pests. Plow your herbs into the soil in fall when they begin to die. The green manure of this plant material will attract fungi which in turn will prey on soil pests.

It is an easy matter to plant some of these herbs right alongside the plants you wish to protect. Mints, thyme, rosemary, winter savory, garlic, in fact any of the so called strong herbs will do the trick. Garlic, whose horrendous odor is capable of destroying friendships, is one of the most remarkable herbs. Its bulb contains a strong sulfur compound called allyl sulfide, which has been 95% effective in destroying aphids. Planted between tomatoes it controls cutworms and hornworms. It is great with cabbages, roses, beans and all greens subject to chewing and sucking insects or egg-laying moths.

If you wish to make a spray for your houseplants, here is the formula. Put several garlic cloves in two tablespoons of mineral oil and allow to stand overnight. Put in blender with a tablespoon of fish emulsion and a cup of water. That's it.

Nasturtiums will deter squash bugs if planted around your cucumbers and squash. In fact, a few nasturtium leaves added to soapy water is an excellent spray. Wormwood is another potent insecticide and an excellent spray can be made with its leaves. I have planted marigold seeds for plants I'll use in the greenhouse this winter. And, of course, lots of garlic!

❖

Touching Is an Antidote

Touching! Why are people afraid to touch, to hug, to kiss? Do they think there is something immoral about it? Is a cold handshake more to their liking? Is it enough for the lonely, the sad, the sick human being who craves the pressure of the arms of a friend upon their shoulders, or a hug, or a kiss?

The men of many countries greet their male friends with a kiss on both cheeks, and they bestow a tender kiss on the fingers of their female companions. Are we so cold-blooded or so prim and proper that we deliberately quell the urge to give someone a hug? Perhaps we should hide some of our prejudices under the mattress where they'll warm up a bit.

We have drugs to combat most of our ailments. Exercise to limber up our joints, sleep to recoup our energy, but what do we do with our emotions? Let them build up to a climax of tears and a feeling of abandonment, or do we have a friend who doesn't think that touching belongs only to the ladies of the night? Yes, I'm a toucher, a hugger, a kisser, but isn't every member of the Irish ancestry? Perhaps touching is the antidote we need to get over our fighting sprees!

William Petersen says these words about giving: "We give of ourselves when we give of the heart, ideas, dreams, ideals, projects and poetry."

How can one express such things with a cold handshake? That kind of giving calls for touching, hugging, kissing. Try it. You might be surprised how much happier even the hugger feels.

❖

Color Behavior

So often, I have wondered why color affects the behavior of people. I know why it affects me. I remember a day when I had to give a talk to a group of pharmacists and I wanted to do a good job. But I had dressed in a brown suit. About a mile from home, I turned around and changed into a blue dress. The brown depressed me and I felt I wouldn't do my best. Blue raised my spirits and gave me confidence. I was happy. I like other colors but not with the enthusiasm I have for shades of blue, from the palest baby blue to the magnetic midnight blue of an evening sky. Brown and dark green make me sad. Purple depresses me and red arouses my Irish temper.

I think most people are affected by color. Certainly members of the health team are now very much aware of color influence upon the sick, and have changed the everlasting white of hospital walls into more soothing pastels. Color changes the attitude of sick children and children's wards have been made more attractive by the use of color. The drab, depressing browns of vehicles such as trains and buses have been replaced with something a little more gay.

Winston Churchill, who enjoyed his painting as relief in times of war stress once said, "I cannot pretend to be impartial about colors. I rejoice with the brilliant ones. When I get to heaven, I mean to spend a considerable amount of time of the first million years in painting and forget the poor brown colors. But then I shall require a still gayer palette than I get here below. I expect orange and vermillion will be the darkest and dullest colors upon it, and beyond them there will be a whole range of wonderful new colors which will delight the celestial eye."

Why did I think of color? Look at the glory around us!

❖

Chervil

There's a patch of beautiful green in my herb garden, and although it is infringing on my asparagus bed, I am loath to redirect it, for chervil isn't the easiest herb to persuade to stay with us. A biennial, it drops its seeds when fully matured and surprises us with a second crop in late September, when other greens have adopted a garment of brown.

Chervil, with its anise-caraway flavor, can perform wonders with so many foods. A famous continental soup is made with chervil and many other soups are flavored with it. Its chopped leaves are added to salads and it gives a distinctive flavor to all kinds of dressings.

When chopped chives and chervil are kneaded into sweet butter, a gourmet treat is created.

Although chervil has never had much of a medicinal reputation, beyond the ancient use of the roots as a soothing, warming dish for chilled stomachs, it was also used by some of my ancestors for pleurisy. It is considered to be a cousin of the parsleys, and because its flavor is so tender, it should be used more generously. Try it in salads, sprinkled over eggs whether they be scrambled, fried or poached. Marry them to potato salad whether hot or cold. One of our popular herbalists recommends it be added to spinach soup, all egg dishes, French dressing, fish, and butter sauces for chicken.

My specialty is good chicken stock with small meat balls and lots of chopped chervil. Anyone can toss a piece of meat on a barbecue—there isn't much imagination to that—so why not add a little spice to your cooking and give a spark to your life. If the way to a man's heart is through his stomach—make the way as pleasant as possible.

❖

What Is Beauty?

Yesterday I drove through a fairyland of beauty, a valley filled with the lovely blossoms of Juneberrys in delicate pastel shades and emitting an ethereal fragrance. It was an experience to store in one's memory for the days when happiness seems to have taken a vacation.

I asked myself, "What is beauty?" The rosy hues of sunrise and the brilliant scarlet of sunset, yes, even the ominous clouds preceding a storm. What is lovelier than a rose unfolding on a sunny day, the scarlet of a poppy or the upturned face of a violet.

Are there colors more beautiful than those of a peacock's feather or the green and scarlet of a humming bird? For the beauty of sound, listen to the song of the birds, the gentle wash of running water, distant thunder and the voice of a loved one.

Consider the beauty in the eyes of an aged man when he looks on the face of one he loves, or the devotion in the eyes of a dog. Touch the bark of a birch tree or the soft green of wood mosses.

We can pick beauty out of the past. Music of the masters, books of great writers, paintings of artists who produced priceless treasures. Beauty may fade at times, but it never really leaves us. We just need to use our five senses to appreciate it.

"Beauty is nature's coin, must not be hoarded, but must be current, and the good thereof consists in mutual and partaken bliss." So said Milton. I think I like the sentiment of Keats, "A thing of beauty is a joy forever; its loveliness increases; it will never pass into nothingness."

❖

Alfalfa

When we see a field of alfalfa, we just naturally associate it with cattle. But did you know that the Chinese eat the leaves of alfalfa as a vegetable. Alfalfa isn't just fodder for animals. It is mainly a leguminous plant, much like peas and beans, however, the leaves are eaten rather than the seeds alone. Alfalfa was one of the first known herbs, used over two thousand years ago by the Arabs, but it is only recently that we have rediscovered its valuable properties.

Alfalfa is a rich source of potassium, magnesium, phosphorus and calcium. It is a good remedy for blood pressure, for it contains all the necessary elements for softening hard arteries. Its rich iron content renders it a specific remedy for anemia, and its calcium content prevents dental problems. Many who are looking for youth and longevity would probably find it in a tea made from the dried green leaves of this wonder herb. (Guess I'll buy some right now!)

In England this herb is known as Lucerne and as Buffalo Herb in parts of this country. Alfalfa is believed to have originated in Southwestern Asia and historical accounts show it was first cultivated in Iran; but in 1854 it was brought to San Francisco and from there spread rapidly over the Western United States.

In the form of silage, Alfalfa Hay is fed to dairy cows, beef cattle, sheep, hogs, horses, and poultry. It is also an excellent honey crop for bees and it is used to increase the vitamin content of prepared foods.

Alfalfa production in the United States averages over eighty five million tons a year. The most important alfalfa producing states are California, Idaho, Washington, South Dakota, Kansas and Nebraska.

It has been found that the green leaf of the Alfalfa contains eight essential enzymes: Lipaze, a fat-splitting enzyme; amylase, which acts upon starches; coagulase, which coagulates milk and acts upon blood clotting; emulsin acts upon sugar; invertase which converts cane sugar into dextrose, and there are other enzymes which aid digestion. Alfalfa sprouts contain more protein than other grains. However, it is the Chlorophyll which gives Alfalfa so much healing quality.

❖

Letter Writing, a Lost Art?

The morning had been rough, with more than the usual small jobs to take care of, and I felt very much in need of a "lift." That was when I decided to find out what the mailman had brought.

Under the usual "throwaways" was a letter from an old friend, a letter filled with happy memories of days we had both spent together. There was so much light and life in those two pages and they renewed my enthusiasm and humor. Why does letter writing seem to be an almost lost art? It is such a powerful tool, why don't we cultivate it to greater perfection?

One of the most pleasant hours I ever spent, was reading a number of letters written by some of our great statesmen. They were masters in the art of letter writing. Not always were they flattering to the recipients, I am sure, but because of their subtle artistry, no one could be too offended. Letter writing is such a wonderful way to say the things that are deep in the heart of a person. They are not words printed on a card to please the eyes, but words that can lighten the burdens of life, and brings smiles to the weary ones.

An unexpected letter to an old friend or a faithful customer could do much to create a warmth where there was indifference. Letters of appreciation to those who work for us, not only in our own organizations, but to those men and women in government who we feel are serving us diligently, would, surely, give them a much needed lift.

As letter writers we are getting lazy for we let the greeting card do all our thinking for us. It tells of our deep sympathy for the sorrowing, our joy for the graduating student, expresses our happiness to the birthday child and the new bride. Does it ever say the things you have in your heart? No! There is great art in letter writing and it is still a very powerful tool.

Now, I'll go and write a letter to one of my old friends.

❖

Witches Garden

Sometime ago, my daughter gave me a book entitled "A Witches Guide To Gardening." Over a cup of tea I have been reading and chuckling. "Everyone knows that senna is a cure for toothache, that the elm tree is magic protection against thunderstorms and marigolds against witchcraft."

"But do you know how to fix a love potion, or how to scare away witches and curses and how to please good fairies?" Isn't that quite a preface to a book on gardening? But there are some delightful scraps of information as one turns the pages. For instance, the marigold, which at one time was associated with the Virgin Mary, was also considered especially effective in restoring eyes to health; but it must be taken only when the moon is in the sign of the Virgin.

"Blackberries are a fruit in which the devil takes a personal interest." They must never be picked after October first as he spits on them after that date. Parsley must always be sown on Good Friday, for this is the only day the health-giving plant can keep the devil in check, and for times the amount required must be sown to allow the devil his quota!

And this was the parsley payoff. "On no account must it ever be transplanted, or dreadful disaster will overtake the household. It must always be planted by the mistress of the house; if any other woman in the house plants it, she will become pregnant."

Despite that warning, I plant eight ounces of parsley seed each year. I wonder what's wrong with me!!

❖

Carrots

"I like cauliflower," said one of my finicky eating friends, "but when you find out what country invented carrots, ask them please, to take them back." One would really suppose he didn't like carrots! And why not, for they are beneficial vitamin-wise. A carrot is one of the most versatile and flavorsome of all vegetables. So, my carrot despising friend, allow me to explain.

The carrot gets its name from the Latin word carola, and it has been known since ancient times and is believed to have originated in Afganistan. Our common carrot is called the Mediterranean type because it has long been known in Mediterranean countries and was probably developed there from Asia Minor.

As is true in a number of other vegetables, it seems that the first interest in carrots as food, developed from their supposed medicinal value. Greek physicians around the first century of our era wrote of carrots and their value as a stomach tonic. Are we amused by the ancients attaching so much importance to the medicinal value of the carrot? Our nutrition experts know the value of carrots for their vitamin A and carotene content. The American Indians certainly discovered the value of this much maligned vegetable and they took up carrot culture in a big way. So, my carrot-despising friend, how about trying a few new ways of preparing this very desirable vegetable.

For instance, a carrot likes stimulating company, so why not combine them with mushrooms, celery, green peppers, or perhaps with your favorite vegetable. Or, slice them, cook them and fold into a good cream sauce, put them into a casserole, top with bread crumbs and grated cheese and put under the broiler to brown. This next one is my favorite. Six large carrots, scrubbed but not peeled, slice very thin. In a saucepan melt two tablespoons of butter, add one tablespoon of finely chopped onion, saute for one minute. Add pepper, salt, paprika and lemon juice. Cook quickly.

Carrots! I love 'em!

Vitamin B12

"How can I get vitamin B12?" I was asked a while ago. Vitamin B12, which is a water-soluble substance, is essential for longevity. It cannot be made synthetically but must be grown, like penicillin, in bacteria or molds. Animal protein is almost the only source in which B12 appears naturally in foods in substantial amounts. Liver is the best source: kidney, muscle meats, fish and dairy products are other good sources.

After B12 is absorbed into the body it is transported into the bloodstream and taken to various tissues. The highest concentrations of this vitamin are found in liver, kidneys, heart, pancreas, testes, brain, blood and bone marrow. These body members are all related to the red blood cell formation. People deficient in B12 usually lack one or more gastric secretions necessary for its absorption. Many people lack the ability to absorb it at all. Absorption of B12 appears to decrease with age and with iron, calcium, and B2 deficiencies, and the use of laxatives depletes the storage of B12.

Symptoms of vitamin B12 deficiency may take five or six years to appear. A deficiency begins with changes in the nervous system such as soreness and weakness of the legs and arms, diminished reflex response and sensory perception, difficulty in walking and speaking (stammering), and jerking of limbs. It has also been found to cause a certain type of brain damage which may be detected by the following symptoms: sore mouth, numbness or stiffness, a feeling of deadness, shooting pains, needles and pins, or hot and cold sensations. A deficiency also manifests itself in nervousness, neuritis, unpleasant body odor, and difficulty in walking.

The Medical Press reported remarkable results in the treatment of osteoarthritis, a degenerate joint disease, and osteoarthritis, a softening of the bone, with B12. It also provides relief from fatigue, nervous irritability, mild impairment in memory, ability to concentrate, mental depression, insomnia and lack of balance. Good old B12!

❖

Potpourri

I have always been interested in potpourris, and for many years I have added fragrant blossoms and essential oils to a large vessel of the fragrant potpourri which fills the house with memories of roses, violets, rosemary and jasmine, for these were my favorite blossoms.

I have been stirring this aromatic mixture this morning and my hands would give joy even to a naughty child waiting to be spanked.

There are many mixtures, all of which make a good potpourri. Always use a container you can seal tightly. I started my potpourri with the following items; a quart each of rose petals, lilac, jasmine, tuberose, rosemary and patchouli. Be sure the petals are dry, then add three tablespoons of ground orrisroot, this is very necessary, and then add the essential oils. I use a teaspoonful of oil of rose geranium, rose, bergamot, and orange. The fragrance of this mixture will increase as time goes on and one can make many beautiful gifts with a small amount of the mixture.

Today we have to rely on synthetic oils which do not last like the essential oils. Until synthetics came into use, it took one ton of roses to make ten ounces of natural oil. Twenty-five tons of violets were required to make a single ounce of the natural oil, but it was never possible to obtain essential oil of lilac until it was made by synthesis, similarly, there was no lily-of-the-valley perfume until it was made synthetically.

If you are fond of the fragrance of many spices to be found around the kitchen, remember that there is also a potpourri made of these condiments and it is really good. Dried basil leaves, caraway, cloves, ginger, marjoram, nutmeg, peppermint, pimento, and thyme.

Put them all in a bag and hang them in your kitchen when your dinner smells bland.

I remember a story I was told about cloves when I was a child. Cloves were known in China before Christ, and it was the custom for court officials to hold a clove in their mouths before addressing their soverign so that their breath might be sweet!

❖

Plants, Living Together

No one could ever convince me that plants are inanimate, senseless, no-feeling-at-all objects. They can be as antagonistic as a sixteen-year-old adolescent and as tempermental as Madame Callas, the singer. You may think you own them, but they own you, and if you don't watch out they'll dictate your every move.

I well remember when I baby-sat some African violets for a friend during the winter. I placed them in a group in a sunny window. A few days later I removed one and placed it in the center of the dining table. In less than 24 hours those beautiful blue blossoms began to fall off and the leaves began to droop. All at once it was ugly so I put it back with the rest of the clan, and in a few hours it began to perk up. I imagine the conversaton between those temperamental plants went something like this, "What makes her think we can be parted from each other. Bet she won't try that again." And I didn't.

Perhaps one of the most flagrant demonstrations that plants have feeling, likes and dislikes is something that happened several years ago but which has remained in my memory. Removing plants from the greenhouse to grace the patio, I placed a huge Boston fern behind a varigated impatiens; I also put another impatiens some distance away with nothing more than white petunias for company. In a few hours, the impatiens backed by the Boston fern, dropped all its rosie petals and the beautiful varigated leaves hung limply over the pot. I examined it for slugs and other noxious varmints, but all was well. Still it continued to droop...not to die, but just look miserable, while its counterpart with the white petunias was a thing of joy. Late that summer I brought the Boston fern indoors and left the impatiens outdoors expecting it would soon expire. Late that afternoon I realized how little I knew of plant behavior—the impatiens that looked so sick in the morning, had brightened up to a "take me indoors condition."

Guess we are never too old to learn.

❖

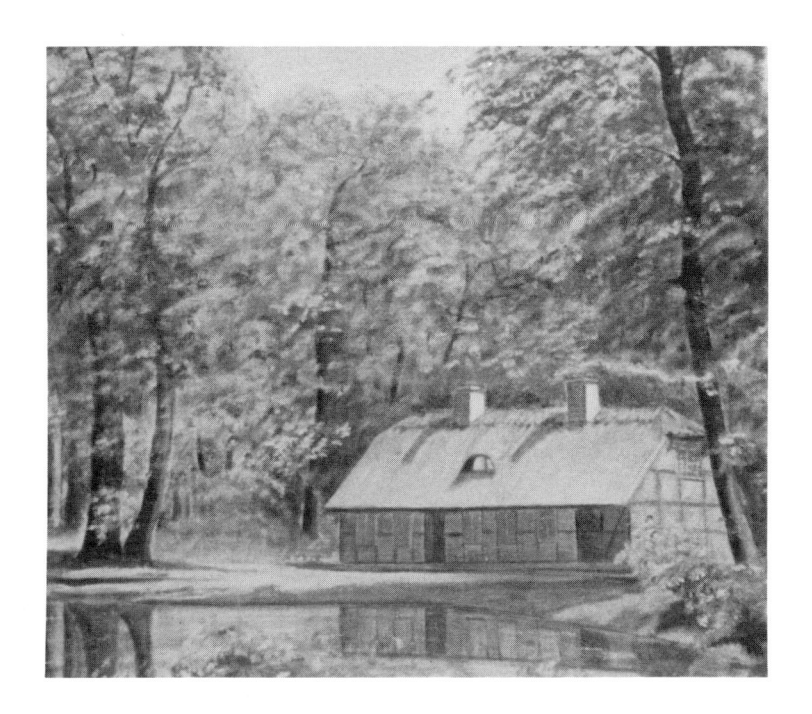

Just Sounds

The sounds of summer! The eerie, almost ominous stillness that precedes the onset of a heavy rain storm. The mournful call of a bird disturbed in the night by a marauding hawk.

The drone of a plane as it moves across the dark, blue velvet of the western sky and the yelping of young coyotes in a nearby ravine.

Cautious animal sounds as they tread the undergrowth of the woods and the soft lap-lap of lake water.

From the woods, a cavern of shadow laced with moonlight, came the snort of a deer tinged with anger.

The day had been warm and voluptuous, and nothing seemed to crave sleep, for across the horizon, like a high wind in pine trees came the deep, mournful sound of a cow's lowing.

Morning came on crimson feet and bird-song filled the land. Early morning breezes went soughing through the trees awakening lazy birds whose singing period was finished for the season. Chipmunks chased each other, their feet making scratching sounds along the bark of the trees. In the distance a dog barked greetings to the new day and a loon flapped its wings on the water of the lake as it prepared for flight.

An insect symphony of cicadas and crickets, interspersed with the humming of honey bees, brought music to a new day.

Just sounds. Bits of melody to those who listen. Parts of mother earth. Companionship and a feeling of not being alone in the world. The sights, the smells, the sounds—all for those who are fortunate enough to stand still and listen. The things that are free—and so very beautiful.

❖

Jewel Weed

The poison ivy plants are flourishing again and I am reminded that it is time for the jewel weed to be budding. Jewel weed is the answer to poison ivy rash which annoys many people in summertime. This delicate wild flower contains napthoquinone, an ingredient which is used in many pharmaceutical preparations, made to relieve the itch of poison ivy.

Jewel weed, or touch-me-not as it is often called, belongs to the impatiens family. This plant grows in moist places; it is a tender, tall-growing annual with butter-yellow flowers, and light green leaves which are very juicy. When the flowers die and the seeds appear, they will shoot from their pods with a snapping sound.

To make a decoction for ivy poisoning, cut the stems and flowers of the jewel weed into small pieces, pour boiling water over and simmer until the juice is extracted and is concentrated. It is of no use to keep the liquid in the refrigerator, but if it is poured into ice trays, frozen and stored in the freezer in plastic bags, it is always available when needed. Rub an ice cube over affected parts, or allow ice to melt and just use the liquid.

The early settlers learned from the Indians how to use jewel weed. They used it for preventing and curing poison ivy rash, but also for itchy scalp, athlete's foot and many other types of fungus infections. One of my old encyclopedia states that the juice of the jewel weed, when mixed with lard is a cure for hemorrhoids. It is also reported to be effective in the removal of warts, corns and similar growths on the skin. Some of these valuable herbs were in use as long ago as 2500 B. C. Perhaps the ancient physicians and philosophers could teach us a few things today that we seem unable to cope with.

❖

Medicinal Plants along the Road

I am always amazed as I walk through the woods and along the roads, at the number of medicinal plants I find. The jewel weed is a foot high and already buds are formed. The medicinal values of this plant are most welcome, particularly to those who get dermatitis from poison ivy. It cures a poison ivy rash in a hurry, but the Indians used jewel weed to treat itch, unhealthy scalp, athletes foot and many kinds of dermatitis of fungus origin.

This morning I found a patch of good, healthy alehoof, or what I call gill or ground ivy, its pale blue flowers giving away its location. I have seen many ulcerated legs completely cured with this lowly, creeping plant, and our forebears made a tea of equal parts of gill and parsley to relieve kidney problems. Milkweed is pushing its lovely green through the earth, and in retrospect, I smell the fragrant blossoms, but it is the juice, the podophyllum, which is used to eliminate warts, ringworm and ordinary sores. The young buds are also good to eat but must be treated properly to eliminate the bitter principle.

Witch hazel bushes are healthy and full of new shoots. Is there a more versatile plant than this? As an astringent, after shave lotion, dandruff remedy, wet applications for sprains and small blood clots, and for soothing tired, inflamed eyes.

Pretty soon the woods roads will be alive with the golden blossoms of St. Johns Wort, which I remember as herb tea for the tummyache. Stinging nettles instead of sulphur and molasses, and a wonderful nettle beer that really clears the complexion. And if you are tired of all this, gather a few leaves of catnip, pour over one cup of boiling water, sip and sleep—but be sure the cat is outdoors.

"*The Lord has created medicines out of the earth and he that is wise will not abhor them.*" —Ecclesiasticus 38-4.

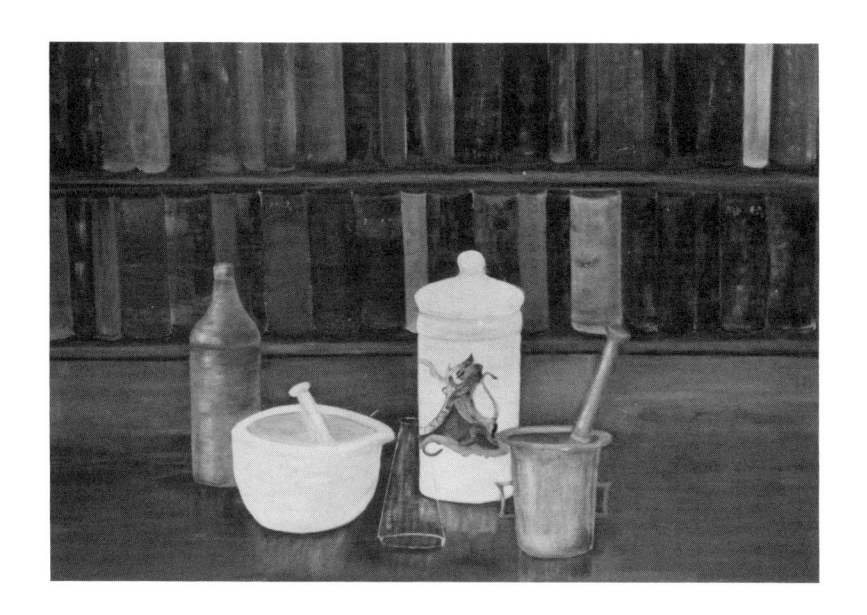

The Pharmacist

Drug stores no longer double as social centers and ice cream parlors, and friendly pharmacists may seem to be an endangered species. That is the opinion of a group of California nutritionists. Here is the advice of a pharmacist.

If you need prescriptions fairly often, try to have one pharmacist fill them all. A good pharmacist needs to get to know you. If your pharmacist is conscientious, he/she will keep your "drug" file on record—a confidential rundown of medications prescribed, food and drug allergies, and your doctor's name and address. If you are seeing more than one doctor, the pharmacist can spot drug incompatibilities they, or you, may not be aware of. Even if you are only buying aspirin, you may need expert advice. Shop for a pharmacist who's willing to keep you, and be sure he/she is available, not only for filling prescriptions but for answering questions.

Suppose you didn't quite understand what your doctor said. Are you sure whether to take the drug before, with, or after meals? If you miss a dose, is it advisable to take two? Should you take all the medication, or quit when you feel better? Your pharmacist may know, or at least be willing to telephone your doctor to find out. Remember these men and women don't study drugs in just one semester. Drugs, their origin, their therapeutic effect on the body and all their side effects—and there are plenty—take years of study. When a pharmacist becomes registered with the state Pharmaceutical board, you may be sure he/she knows their job thoroughly.

Lots of adults can't deal with child-proof containers. Don't be shy about admitting it and asking for a different kind of cap, as long as there are no children in your home. If the print on the label is hard to read, say so. A good pharmacist will package the prescription to suit you. For example, he/she will provide different colored containers for multiple medications so that you don't confuse them.

Depend upon your pharmacist. You'll be happy you did.

❖

Walking and Yoga

I was with a few friends a while ago when exercise was the subject of discussion, and I was asked what kind, if any, exercise I indulged in. Of course, I could have mentioned the twenty odd times a day I rush across two rooms to open the door for an in-and-out energetic Dalmation dog. Perhaps I should have demonstrated the stretching exercises enjoyed (?) when I hang the laundry on the clothes line, or the spontaneous isometrics when the hammer I am using misses the wood and plays havoc with my thumb. But the question was serious so I spoke of my daily walk, for I believe walking is the best exercise for one who has enjoyed all the dancing gymnasts of a century almost, and wishes to finally settle down to something more dignified.

Walking not only exercises the body but the senses of smell, touch, hearing and seeing, for in a gym, how can one smell the blossoms of a trailing arbutus, touch the bark of a birch, hear the song of birds or see the glorious clouds. Besides that, walking uses 216 calories per hour. It also helps the entire system function better. The metabolism is increased while walking, thus fat is burned up and weight loss promoted. Blood pressure, blood cholesterol, and sugar levels tend to fall. Walking builds up the heart muscle and keeps the arteries clear and elastic. Walking helps increase the oxygen supply to the blood, thus bringing more oxygen to the heart. It also increases the capacity of the lungs making more oxygen available to the circulatory system.

There are many other types of exercise, most of which are beneficial. Yoga, for instance, can be practiced by people of all ages, but should be taught by an experienced teacher. Yoga relieves the body of tension, gives elasticity to the spine, tones flabby muscles and improves poor posture. Don't forget skiing, golf, tennis and skating as well as dancing, stretching and jogging. Go to it and stir up your tired senses!

❖

The Versatile Vinegar

I have just finished swabbing an insect bite with vinegar to kill the sting, and I am wondering how many times I have used vinegar for other things. A wee bit in the bread dough to keep it from molding during hot weather; in cauliflower to keep down the odor while cooking; and in the water in which I poached my morning egg.

I also use vinegar to clean windows, and when I have a copper-cleaning streak a paste made with salt, flour and vinegar, and even my mother-in-law (if I had one) would declare I was a good housekeeper. For most of us, vinegar is a household staple. We need it for salad dressings, and for canning pickles, etc., but vinegar is also a medicine, a deodorant, a cosmetic, and, mixed with water, soda or alcohol it makes cleaning solutions for almost dozens of purposes.

As a young apprentice pharmacist, I had a Frenchman for a boss who would periodically order me to make Vinaigre des quatre voleurs, which was vinegar with oils of lavender, rosemary, lemon, cloves and others which I have forgotten. This preparation was known over two hundred years ago as Vinegar of the Four Thieves, because it was alleged to have been used as a prophylactic against the plague in Marseilles by four thieves who robbed the dead and the dying.

Vinegars have been used since the days of Hippocrates. Medicated vinegars are the solutions of the active principals of drugs in diluted acetic acid, which is not only a good solvent but also a good antiseptic.

Have you ever made a batch of cookies that called for buttermilk? You have no buttermilk, so use a dash of vinegar and there is your buttermilk. Sour cream can be made with sweet cream and a dash of vinegar. And if you are fed up with ants, try washing countertops and other ant-interested places with half water and half vinegar.

The versatile vinegar. *What would we do without it?*

❖

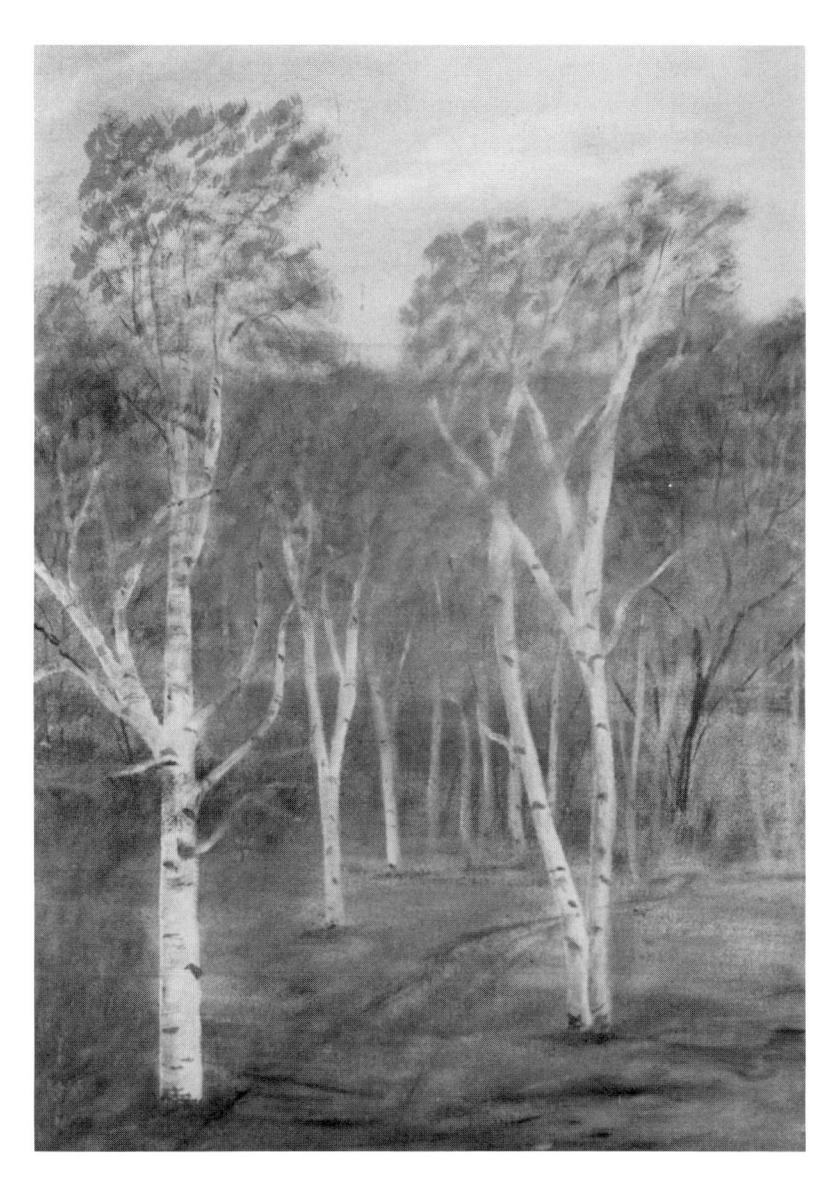

Late Summer

    There's something sad about summer's ending. Bird song is stilled, the chirp of crickets has a lazy meter; prairie asters lie like a shroud of mist across the fields, while brighter New England asters, hang their dusty heads disconsolately along the roadside, and there's an odor of decaying vegetation in the air.

The brilliant plumage of summer birds is seldom seen, while blue jays, chickadees and nuthatches are back at the feeding stations reminding us that they intend to be freeloading again this winter.

Choke cherries and pin cherries hang heavy with juice pulling down the branches, begging to be picked. Squirrels eye the hazel nuts which are just about ripe, while chipmunks begin hoarding acorns for winter use.

The chaste white blossoms of wintergreen are giving way to scarlet berries and partridge berries, bright spots of ruby jewels, brighten the floor of the woods.

Bracken, brown as burnished leather, is beautiful even as it dies. There's a sluggishness to the sound of the river, like a tired old man whose energy has evaporated with summer's heat.

Late summer sadness? Yes! But look upward to where the scarlet of maple leaves, the gold of birch and the copper tones of oak bring promise of a glorious autumn. Each season brings its beauty with colors painted by the Master artist.

——— ❖ ———

Geraniums

Late last fall I made cuttings of many geraniums, hoping they would be ready to bloom by spring, but today I have a large bowl filled with bright red, pink and white blossoming geraniums, a joyful sight on a dull day. I think they are the most democratic of all flowers. So homey in their gay peasant colors, and they are at ease on the roof garden of a city penthouse or in the windowboxes of exclusive clubs. They are equally natural to suburban or small-town homes and seaside cottages and they are just right on anyone's windowsill. A kitchen with geraniums advertises itself as a friendly, tidy, busy place that invites visitors.

The tiny, velvety, four-petal flowerettes of the geranium make a staunch clump of color on a sturdy stem graced with abundant leaves which look like little frilled doll aprons.

We seldom think of geraniums as having a fragrance--at least not an outstanding fragrance. But they do, and their fragrance is what is known as "whole" fragrance, for not only the blossoms, but the leaves and stems are used extensively in perfumes and especially in scenting hand soaps and it blends well with rose and oriental perfumes. The fragrance of geranium, seeming to contain within itself the vibrant color of the flower, is perfectly suited to soaps which just ought to smell crisp, clean, and colorful.

Geraniums are cultivated for the perfumer in many parts of the world—Reunion, Algeria, Spain, Russia, Southern France, and the Belgian Congo. Reunion alone produces almost 200,000 pounds of oil of geranium a year.

Geraniums were introduced to Algeria about 80 years ago. Here the natives work under the blistering sun, cutting the plants and carrying them to the stills.

You may have always thought of geranium as a flower fragrance, but the leaves and stems are the valuable part. I just love them for being so humble and so appreciative of even a little care.

❖

Ambergris

As I watched the rescuing of whales in the North seas, I wondered, if among those great animals there might be a sperm whale. This is the great sea animal that produces the most valuable item used in the manufacture of fine, expensive perfumes—Ambergris. It is the sperm whale alone which gives us Ambergris, that most valuable and important of all fixatives. What is the origin of this extraordinary stuff that only Mr. Sperm Whale contributes to civilization?

It seems that his particular delicacy is cuttle fish or squids and that, sometimes, his digestive system just can't cope with the intake. So he suffers from indigestion on a large scale and his intestines are irritated, presumably from the horny beaks, so he ejects his dinner. Only one sperm whale among thousands that have been ripped open in great excitement yields this treasure. It might be compared to finding a beautiful pearl in an oyster—only much more so! There are dozens of exciting tales of whalers who think they've found Ambergris, only to be disappointed when they find they have picked up some worthless blubber. Although the professional whaler is the most likely person to find Ambergris, non-whalers have stumbled on it unawares.

The thrilling story is told of some Hawaiian cowboys who had been taking their ponies for a dip when they noticed masses of what they supposed was sponge, which they used to wipe down their animals. Curiosity overcame them and they took a few pieces for someone to examine. When they learned what they had discovered, they dashed back to the spot to retrieve their floating fortune. Most of it had been washed out with the tide, but they salvaged enough for a comfortable living the rest of their lives.

These sea patches of Ambergris may weigh anything from a few ounces to a pound or two, but there have been masses found weighing a hundred pounds or more. One mass weighing two hundred and forty pounds brought the fabulous price of one hundred thousand dollars.

So, if we like good perfume, we had better pray for the sperm whale.

——— ❖ ———

Plants Clean Pollution

Dr. Anthony Nero, a leader of indoor air quality studies at Lawrence Berkley Labs in California, said, "the risks posed by indoor pollutants are in fact comparable in magnitude to those associated with exposure to chemicals or radiation in industrial settings."

Scientists say that polluted rooms cannot be cleaned up by plants alone but a few well-chosen greenery can reduce the levels of some dangerous contaminants. The first results of the new research, announced recently, showed that eight plants tested with benzene, which is known to cause some human cancers, two, the Gerbera daisy and Chrysanthemum, were rated "superior" in removing the pollutant from the experimental chamber.

I was particularly interested to read this because I was given two Gerbera plants a month ago. Their luxuriant foliage and bright flowers are a joy.

In the studies, the leaves of elephant ear, known scientifically as Philodendron, and golden pothos, demonstrated their ability to remove benzene and carbon monoxide from closed chambers. Two kinds of philodendron, elephant ear and heart leaf, were found to absorb large quantities of formaldehyde from the air.

People are constantly exposed to this toxic chemical, which is used in certain foam insulations, plywood, particle board, grocery bags, waxed papers, facial tissues, carpet backing, fire retardants and permanent-press clothing. Aloe Vera proved to be more effective than the others in removing formaldehyde at low concentrations, the scientists said.

I wonder how much Tennyson knew of plant life when he wrote "Flower in the crannied wall, I pluck you out of the crannies, I hold you here, root and all in my hand, little flower - but if I could understand what you are root and all, I should know what God and man is."

❖

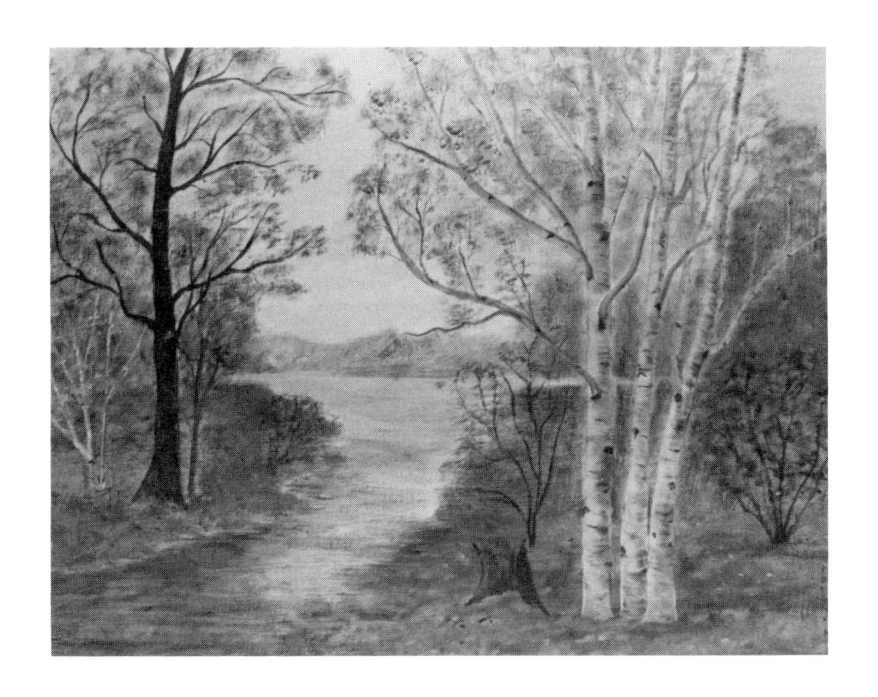

A Summer Morning

There's something magical about a summer morning. To walk in the woods the first hour after dawn, is to gather impressions that will last a lifetime. Everything is dusted with the soft, ethereal pink of dawn light, like the delicate frosting on a cake. Muted rustlings of small animals rustle in the undergrowth; squirrels are casting an inquiring eye on the intruder. Wood thrushes will direct you away from their nesting place. A ruffled grouse, perched on a fallen log will be cleaning his feathers, making ready for a day of exploring.

The floor of the woods will be patterned with dappled sunlight, moving back and forth like weary ballet dancers.

There will be dewdrops clinging to the branches of broken ferns and across the exquisite artistry of a spider's web. Bright spots of blood red wintergreen berries daring to be picked and tasted, peep shyly through the Princess Pines, and the shiny leaves of hepatica vie for prominence with wild geranium and bloodroot.

Green as an Irish meadow are the mosses with their myriads of exquisitely minute flowers, and if you are hungry, wild strawberries are there for the picking. Maybe the birds have left a few fruits on the shadberry trees. Gather a few for your breakfast and enjoy a different taste.

There's a fragrance in early-morning woods. A warm, umberish odor of decaying tree trunks and rotting leaves. The pleasant, almost comforting smell of lichens and mosses, and the occasional waft of balsam fragrance.

Listen! Chickadees, already warning you the day will be warm. The oriole entertaining you with some of earth's most beautiful musical cadences. *Thank God for the magic of a summer morning!*

❖

Herbs Dry and Fresh

Our home is filled with an indescribable fragrance, more delightful to my nostrils than the finest fifty-dollar-an-ounce perfume. Hanging in bunches in an airy passage are freshly gathered Tarragon, Chervil, Orange Mint, Lemon Balm, Winter Savory and Oregano.

In the hydrator lemon thyme is slowly drying and somehow, the entire house is alive. Perhaps it is the thought of the elegant flavors these herbs will add to our menus during the coming year.

Soon after sunrise this morning, I transplanted plants of Basil and I thought of the many legends surrounding this versatile herb. The ancient Greeks believed that Basil wouldn't grow unless planted with curses and abuse. I wonder if my remarks regarding the mosquitoes will assist the growth of the Basil? Basil was first grown in English gardens in the 16th century. It supplied the flavoring for the famous Fetter Lane sausages. I have cut some leaves which I will use on sliced tomatoes which I have sprinkled with oil and vinegar and which will be covered with finely chopped Basil. Oh yes! The rest of the tomatoes will be chopped, simmered for about five minutes, put in the blender with a wee bit of honey and half a cup of chopped Basil. I'll use it as a sauce for egg noodles.

Sweet Basil may be used for many things. It makes excellent herb vinegar and butter. Sprinkled over potatoes and other vegetables, mixed with cream or cottage cheese, and Italian food without the addition of a bit of Basil is as uninteresting as a kiss without a moustache.

❖

A Hint of Autumn

Summer has flaunted her skirts of green,
Skies of blue with clouds serene,
And nights, that hung the stars like lanterns low.

And now, a hint of autumn fills the dawn with mist, reminding us another season nears. September! The bridge we cross into the month of color. Huge crows feed on farmers' fields, while small birds lace telephone wires like jet necklaces. Hawks fly overhead, scavenging the last nests and picking up lazy rodents. Two eagles have been sailing across the blue skies, dropping shadows over sunlit spots of green, and geese rest overnight on the lake. Can summer really be over?

Shadbush in the valley are wearing the plum-red garments of fall, which are almost as beautiful as the blossoms of spring. Maples are already flaunting the scarlets of royalty. Sumac has curled its leaves into patterns of brown and bits of gold are beginning to weave a paisley-like shawl motif across the hills. Blackberries, rose hips, pin and choke cherries are abundant and ready for harvesting, and some of the wild apples provide excellent pectin for jelly making.

Now is the time to make winter bouquets. Beautiful grasses with heavy, ripe heads beckon me as I walk along the road. I'm not sure whether they are bidding me "good morning" or nodding a farewell to Queen Anne's lace. The goldenrod which should never be despised, will dry into a graceful bouquet, and the burnished gold of tansy is ornamental as well as having therapeutic qualities.

Each season has its beauty, and, as we say farewell to the lush greens of summer, we can look ahead with joy to the painting fingers of late September and October and the red and gold beauty of autumn.

Being Liberated

I've just finished reading a book on Women's Lib—whatever that means. My husband asked me if I was interested in being liberated and my answer to him was, that I had always felt liberated.

Until my retirement, I've always had a job, working side by side with men. I felt I knew as much as they did professionally. My salary was the same as theirs, but I was happy to have them beside me, for their arms were stronger than mine and I was glad to have someone who could lift heavy packages or reach for high gallon bottles, and somehow, I never felt inferior to my male colleagues.

Women's Lib! What in heck is it? I'm happy to be a woman. I raised a daughter, so I can cook, keep a house clean, do laundry, and any chore a wife usually does—and I am happy.

So! What am I missing? Apparently, according to some Women's Lib advocates, I'm missing a lot, but by my saintly Aunt Sarah's wig, I'm durned if I know what it is.

I like being a woman. I enjoy having a man open the door for me and seat me at the table. Lordy! How I love having my back rubbed and that recalcitrant zipper on my dress zipped up. I like being presented with fresh flowers in the middle of January and closing my eyes to receive my favorite bottle of perfume when it is neither an anniversary, birthday or Christmas. My heart sings when I am told I am beautiful, even though my mirror snickers. And when I push my fingers through my hair and my husband smiles and puts his arms around me knowing I'm a first class nut—my world just whirls with happiness.

What am I missing? I don't know. I'll brood over it and maybe I'll come up with an answer. But, in the meantime, I'm glad I'm built the way I am, with hills and valleys in the right places; I'm happy I was able to bring a child into the world, that my guardian taught me how to keep a good, clean house; that I learned how to cook, but above all, I'm happy that I have a man who loves me and whom I love.

Women's Lib!!! Phoeee!!!!

❖

Magnificent Autumn

This is the first day of autumn. I went outside before the world had really awakened. Autumn! Capricious artist of the seasons; splashing the world in abandon with colors no artist could possibly copy. Thumbing her nose at summer and flipping her artistic hand at the winter to come.

Small cobwebs festooned the bushes like miniature handkerchiefs and the brief flashes of sunlight turned them to gossamer bits of fancy. The trees were clothed in gypsy colors of scarlet and gold, and they emerged from the mist like ghostly cathedrals.

As morning took over, the birds began their brief autumn song and small animals scuttled to places where acorns lay in abundance along the woods' floor. Red jewels of wintergreen peeped from the bracken that had changed from the green of summer to the burnished leather of autumn. Tiny coral mushrooms, that looked like something to be worn on a white satin blouse, were at the foot of a great oak tree, and a shell-like substance wrapped itself across a fallen log.

There were mosses of every description; the spagnum and pincushion moss predominating—soft as a down pillow. No wonder Lapland mothers line the baby's cradle with this moss. Perhaps they watched the birds as they cushioned their nests with this elegant substance.

I looked across at the distant hills. Sunrise had turned the mist of morning into unbelievable beauty. Like Paisley shawls, the greens, golds, scarlets covered every tree and I felt very humble as I looked at this beautiful world. It keeps my heart young and never allows my dreams to die.

❖

We Are What We Eat

We are what we eat. Isn't that what our grandparents taught us? And they gave us good food. Meat, unembellished with chemicals, vegetables fresh from the garden or root cellar; apples, pears, plums and cherries from the trees, carefully preserved, and greens and wild fruits and berries from the fields and woods. Fish from unpolluted waters and chickens free from hormones to fatten them. We were healthy and without benefit of chemical additives, which was good, for the nearest doctor was miles away, and although there was a hospital, no one seemed to know just where.

Wouldn't you enjoy fresh milk and cream that was real cream? Do you remember when your grandmother made her own cream sauces and didn't use something that came in a package labeled hydrogenated soybean oil, disodium phosphate, citric acid, artifical flavor and coloring, mono and diglycerides?

What happened to good whole wheat grains and unbleached flour and homemade bread spread with freshly churned butter —and don't try selling me that so-called cholesterol-free stuff called Oleo.

Perhaps I am a nut when it comes to nutrition, but as we get older we learn to discriminate, to evaluate right from wrong, true from false, and I believe that the advertising we get regarding the benefit of chemicals and their stabilizing qualities is false. I just wonder what, in our diets, is destroying the natural element in our body which retards the growth of cancer cells?

I also ask myself about the popular chemical monosodium glutamate which creates numbness in certain parts of the body, and which, recently, a group of doctors have found to be the cause of some deaths.

Oh well! I'm hungry. So I'll cook breakfast. A virginal egg and meat cured with sodium nitrate, sodium chloride, sodium phosphate, sodium erythorbate, water—and we call it *bacon*.

❖

Gardening

Have we ever given thought to the therapy of gardening? The joy of seeing the first daffodil in spring, the fragrance of the first rose in summer. The satisfaction of gathering the first radish, chives and lettuce for a refreshing salad without fear of chemical contamination. Have you ever started gardening in the early morning before the insects become active and prepared a bed which will be seeded later in the day. The ozone is fresher, breakfast tastes better and somehow the chores of the day are less pressing.

How does one describe the delight of planting peas and beans and finding tiny greens pushing through the soil days before you expected them. Wasn't it all worth the half hour you spent cultivating in the early morning? Planting potatoes has always intrigued me. One of my earliest girlish memories is of my Irish Granny planting potatoes. She dug up the soil on the potato patch; placed potatoes on top of the ground and covered them with hay and straw. The plants pushed through the covering, did their usual flowering job and formed potatoes. Granny pushed her hand into the straw broke off the potatoes she needed. We had fresh potatoes every day, for there was no pouting on the part of the plant, it just went on producing.

Leeks are another vegetable that fascinated me. Leeks were a must for leek and potato soup and everyone seemed to like the white stem of the vegetable well smeared with butter after they were boiled. Gardeners with a piece of broom handle, would make deep round holes in the soil, place a seed just under the soil after they filled the hole with rich soil and the leek grew fat and white.

What is it that makes gardening so enjoyable? Is it the color and fragrance of the flowers; the taste of good vegetables, or the peace and quiet which eases stress and worry?

"*The kiss of the sun for pardon. The song of the birds for mirth. One is nearer God's heart in a garden than anywhere else on earth.*"

❖

Old Remedies

I'm having fun looking through old recipe books and finding that I still use some of the old remedies some folks consider useless.

For instance, "the fastest way of getting relief after the finger is bruised, or the nail hurt, is to plunge the finger in water as hot as can be borne. By so doing, the nail is softened and allows the blood to pour out beneath it, thereby relieving the pain; the finger may then be wrapped in a bread poultice." My bread poultice consists of bread crumbs softened with hot milk spread on sterile gauze and applied to whatever needs attention.

To remove insects from the ears, put a few drops of warm sweet oil in. To slim yourself, it is necessary to reverse the process by which slim persons become fat. Just diminish the quantities and not eliminate food altogether because that will also reverse a good disposition. (That was one of my Granny's recipes.)

If corns are your bugbear, here's the specific. Wear cotton socks saturated with oil or glycerine and see that it goes between the toes for soft corns. (Try doing that.) For other corns apply fresh every morning, the yeast of small beer spread on a rag. (Where are the home brewers?)

For warts apply bruised ivy leaves daily. Within a fortnight they will drop off! And here's another. Soak a piece of bread in strong vinegar and apply as a poultice.

If aches and pains are not your concern, then think about some garden problems. Slugs, for instance. Put cabbage leaves in the oven until soft, rub with fresh bacon drippings and lay wherever the slugs are. The leaves will soon be covered with snails and slugs. Now let me give you my surefire slug eliminator. Take a piece of soft, porous wood and soak it with beer. Turn the wood, beer side down and just see how these loathsome slugs like their alcohol.

I'm sure you know how much trouble we go to in order to

prevent moth damage. Here's another of Granny's ideas. "Take of pennyroyal a large amount. Crush the leaves and put them in all the places where you keep woolen garments. The odor of it destroys some and drives others away." Watch out moths, here we come!

❖

Talk to Plants

Do I talk to my plants? Of course I do. And they answer. Not in words, of course, but they have the edge on body language. For instance, I have a Dieffenbachia so large, it is trying to push its branches through the porch ceiling. When I water the plant, I always give the beautiful shiny leaves an affectionate pat, which they acknowledge with a shiver of delight. I love plants and flowers and don't wish to be deprived of them during the winter months. The greenhouse is filled with blossoming plants and so is the porch and the front window.

They are kind. They don't criticize me if I am not dressed just right, or if my hair stands on end because I ran my fingers through it while trying to solve a problem. They produce blossoms at the wrong time of the year, when I particularly need a mental pickup.

The Aeschynanthus, which I refer to as the Lipstick Plant, showed me in no uncertain terms that she didn't like her present location, at least not in winter. I moved her to a much warmer spot and in one week she was full of buds, and I swear she wore a smile on every leaf. Of course, plants, like people, can be very temperamental.

One morning, when the sun was shining and every bloom was at its brightest, I lapsed into a bit of Shakespeare. I should have known the Jade plant would object, but she has always been on the tempermental side. Guess I'll just whistle "Dixie" next time I'm near her.

About a year ago, I was given a cactus and was told not to expect blossoms for at least two years. But I wanted to see those beautiful white blooms. Being of impatient Irish ancestry, two years was too long. My Christmas cactus decided to bloom again, the Easter cactus was budding, and the Orchid cactus just thinking about it all. I put them all together and, as an afterthought, added the white flower-bearing new addition. Yes! indeed! Today there is a beautiful, white flower bud on the new cactus. Competition among plants? Certainly.

Humans respond to kindness. So do animals. So why not plants? Just put two plants side by side. Pay particular attention to one of them and neglect the other. Results? One will flourish and the other just pout.

Lordy! Is there someone who will come and converse with my Aspidestra?

❖

Night Sounds

It was the last beautiful evening of October and in the navy blue, diamond-studded sky shone a new moon. I stepped out into the night. Reflected in the lake was the brilliance of Venus, while Neptune rose higher and higher in the sky vying for importance. The night was still. I had the feeling that all life was arrested and at peace, and I listened. Listened to the night sounds, mysterious yet eloquent, elusive but forceful. Full of life in the darkness of night, penetrating but restful. Night sounds! A buck snorted softly below the porch, perhaps testing my friendliness. Across the western hills a coyote gave his peculiar call and was answered from the east with equal enthusiasm. Far down the river, the bugle call of an elk cut through the stillness reminding me that mating season was at hand, and females had better beware or respond.

The song of the stream was solemn and somber, for it was being abandoned by ducks and frogs, and the loneliness of winter was setting in. A tree toad, who had come to life believing summer had postponed her farewell, gave its ventriloquist croak from behind me, then threw the challenge from right beneath my feet. There was a rustle in the leaves and the high-pitched sound of a porcupine made my nerves tingle. A large bird, having escaped the hunter's shells, settled contentedly in the Scotch pine I planted so many years ago, and a night hawk flew perilously close on an investigating forage. Suddenly a brisk wind came hurtling through the Norway pines reminding me of childhood sounds of waves breaking on the coast of the North Sea.

And then all was still. Bright stars, a light mist rising from the lake, the melancholy hoot of an owl. And over all the holy hush of a special bit of God's world.

❖

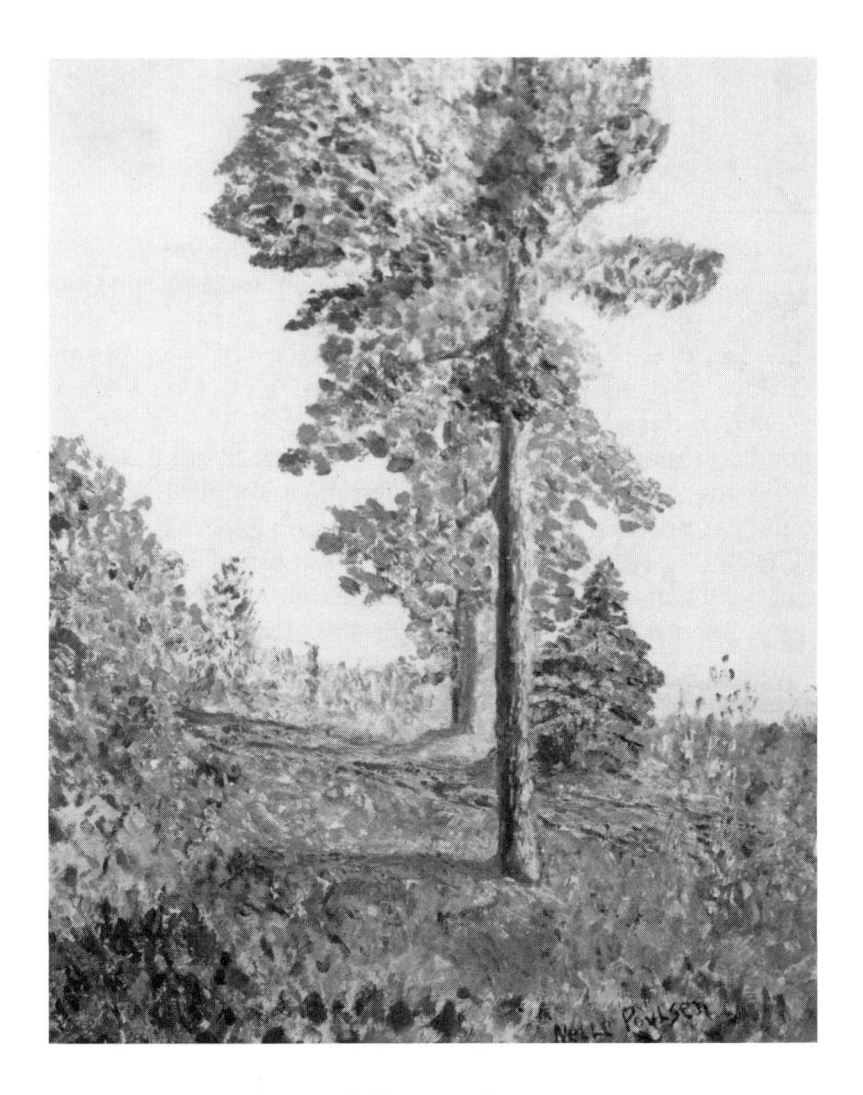

Longfellow's Autumn

    Autumn! Gossamer webs hanging like pristine scraps of chiffon in the spaces of the wire fence. Crows collecting in noisy confusion arguing about the best way to fly to southern climes, while scores of small birds rest quietly on the power lines, symmetrically lined up like agate stones on a necklace. Inquisitive chipmunks wondering if it might not be wise to hibernate, and black squirrels asking whatever happened to summer. Gone are the hummingbirds, and stilled is the cry of the cardinal from a nearby copse. Beautiful formations of Canada geese fly across the lake, then turn about to settle on the water till dawn. Loons are sounding their last hurrah and the lone swan who has lived all summer at the mouth of the river has decided to leave us.

But—the saucy chickadees are back and the shy nuthatch is practicing running backwards on the oak tree; blue jays and hungry grosbeaks are hovering around the empty feeders asking that they be cleaned and filled, and so life goes on in birddom.

In the woods, amongst the burnished bracken green mosses and the scarlet of wintergreen berries, rosy apples, like scarlet bouquets, hang on the wild trees, an alien spot among the golds, reds and copper of the trees, and the last of the mushrooms pop up from the damp earth. The distant hills carry the colors of beautiful Paisley shawls flaunting brilliant colors among the muted greens, and gossamer clouds, scuttled by soft breezes bespeak a summer gone.

Longfellow's definition of Autumn was as follows: "*Magnificent autumn! He comes not like a pilgrim, clad in russet weeds; not like a hermit, clad in gray; but like a warrior, with the stain of blood on his brazen mail. His crimson scarf rent; his scarlet banner dripping with gore; his step like a flail on the threshing floor.*"

❖

Juniper

Down below our front window is a large Juniper bush. It has been loaded with berries, but most of them are gone. I watched a blue jay filling his tummy with the ripe fruit and I remembered that juniper berries are an essential ingredient in gin. So! I became curious, wondering how a tipsy blue jay would act when the juniper oil hit his equilibrium. I guess he's a hardened boozer for he is still hopping around and seems to have control of everything.

Juniper berries are too pungent for human taste until they are dried when they can be used for cooking. They remove the strong flavor of game and give food an interesting flavor. Juniper berries are an inseparable part of gin and they were first used by the 17th century nobleman, the Comte de Moret, son of the French king Henry IV. The very name "gin" comes indirectly from juniper berries, for the French name for gin was genievre.

The juniper tree and berry have long been associated with the protection of people. It is said that when the Virgin Mary and Jesus were trying to escape from the punishment of King Herod by fleeing into Egypt, they hid behind the spreading branches of the juniper and were saved. And Elijah, the prophet while escaping from the Wicked queen Jezebel, wife of Ahab, was protected by an angel when he slept under a juniper in the wilderness. The Romans burned juniper trees to protect themselves from harm and Virgil, the Latin poet, instructs "But learn to burn within your sheltering rooms, sweet juniper."

If you are making a pot roast try adding about ten juniper berries that have been crushed to release the fragrance. But do gather them before the birds discover your treasure.

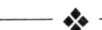

❖

The Brewhouse

I've been going back through the years of my memories and trying to find out what made my ancestors so vigorous: my handsome Scotch-Irish grandfather, who, at 78 years of age, faced the day at 5:30 each morning to attend to his engineering projects; on the other side of the family was Granny: Irish, energetic, with a scintillating wit and a delight in just plain living.

Why? That is what I have been asking myself and this is what I came up with. They brewed! That's right—they brewed! Yeast, malt, hops and demerara sugar. Beer! That's what it was—beer, loaded with vitamin B. They had their brewhouses apart from the house proper. They did their laundry there, too, but it was primarily used for beer making, so it was called the Brewhouse. Yeast, malt, and hops are all loaded with vitamin B, the vitamin that gives us energy and makes us vitally alive.

I never saw anyone in a state of pixilation from drinking this brew, although it was the beverage preferred at "elevenses," midday dinner and high teas. The old folk put a hot poker in a pitcher of the brew and sipped it slowly before they retired—and they slept. No tranquilizer or sedatives, just a pitcher of poker-heated brew, and next morning, free of headaches, they went to work. Of course, we had the teetotalers who looked askance at the drinkers of homebrew, so—they brewed their own. Stinging nettles, gathered by the bushel, boiled and strained into a keg, with lemon slices, demerara sugar and— Lordy!—balm from the top of the working beer of the despised beer drinkers! How else could the nettle beer be persuaded to work? I've never been really sure, but I'll bet all the tea in China there was more than a scrap of intoxication in them there nettles!

Monday was bread-making day and balm was used instead of the yeast we use today, and I've seen many a housewife spoon the bubbly balm into her mouth never knowing how much of her energy came from that effervescing brown substance.

Pancakes and muffins were put to rise the night before, all laced with a bit of balm and cooked on the griddle for breakfast. Ah! There were, of course, those worst of all infidels, who never attended church except for weddings and funerals, but who gathered the wild damson plums from the hedgerows and the purple elderberries which rubbed elbows with the hawthorn. All this, while neighbors prayed for the redemption of their sins (the sins of the beer brewers). Winemakers! Wine worked with the blessed balm from the nettle brewers: the teetotalers, who cheerfully partook of the beverage at weddings and wakes—but that was a different matter. Yeast, balm, vitamin B and some of my Granny's homebrew! Who needs drugs to give them pep? And before I begin to drool, I'll go make a cup of tea!

❖

Healing with Herbs

There is a revived interest in the natural healing power of herbs. Perhaps it is because of the rising cost of man-made medications. The Bible tells us that God "gave every herb for meat" but did not include directions and dosage, and that is what disturbs me.

The European herbalists, and they are numerous, were required to have knowledge of medical material and toxicology, and as I remember, detailed instructions came with every purchase of herbs. As a pharmacist interested in herbs, and with a clientele of customers from the old countries, I carried all kinds of herbs—everything from Buchu to wormwood. They came from a well-known herb house in New York and were packaged in small square boxes with full directions clearly printed on each box. There was safety in such purchases, but today there are indications that some people ignore the fact that there is no truth in "if a little does a good job, a lot more will do better."

There are some excellent herb houses in this country and they are prepared to give directions and dosages, and in many cases they warn customers regarding overdosing, so be on the safe side. Two or three leaves of catnip infused in hot water is a great soporific and will ensure one a good night's sleep, but an overdose is hallucinogenic and could push you into kingdom come before you are ready. Tansy is good—or bad—for worms, but if a great bellyache is what you are looking for, just double the dose.

Because an elderly woman in Derbyshire, England, discovered years ago that a pinch of foxglove leaves relieved her heart pains is no reason to think it will help you. That is why the pharmacologist made digitalis, a product which must be taken with caution and carefully prescribed by a physician.

The Aztec Indians know all about the healing art of herbs, but how do you think they acquired this knowledge? By trial and error and there were many errors and many lives lost. Take care and live.

❖

Walking

Wherever you live, walking is beautiful. Walking is a love affair with life. I have walked in the city, along the seashore, over the heather-covered moors of Yorkshire, the deserted castle grounds of Ireland and our beloved north woods.

I have walked in a winter fantasy of trees filigreed in silver, last fall's apples varnished in gold in the early morning sunlight with the snow lavishly scattering her diamonds at my feet. A while ago, as I walked in the early evening, a bird followed me flying from tree to tree and scolding me with a raucous cry—that is, until I began to whistle, when he probably thought he had encountered an unusually large member of his species.

When things go wrong and anger creeps in, try taking a good brisk walk. It beats throwing dishes and speaking ugly words, and it's amazing how quickly calm takes over. A walk is no further away than your doorstep and all you need are comfortable, flat shoes and light warm clothing.

If insomnia is bugging you, try taking a walk in the moonlight. Listen to the quiet, and to the night sounds, muted, mysterious, filled with promise of a good tomorrow. Let the petty irritations of the day melt into those fantastic shadows created by moonlight.

You are alone with your thoughts, soliloquizing with your Creator, the cobwebs of your mind blowing away, large problems unraveling like silk. You will feel a gentle alchemy taking place within your mind and will become more in tune with yourself and others and infinitely more aware of God as the Creator of life.

Walk to live—and to learn to love.

❖

Irish Moss

'Well, at least it contains a bit of old Ireland' I muttered as I read the list of the contents of a can of food I thought of buying. Yes, the item for thickening was Irish Moss, known to the food industry as Carrageen. My memory went sliding back, remembering all the old stories I had heard through the years about Irish Moss.

During the potato famine of the mid-19th century, thousands of beleaguered Irish saved themselves from starvation by eating the bushy seaweed known as Irish Moss. They were following the example of many generations of hungry poor folk in their own land and other lands that border the North Atlantic Ocean. It is an example that has been followed by many since, when hard times have pressed.

In more bounteous times, the same humble seaweed has served as an effective laxative and as a home remedy for sore throats and chapped skin. It is also commonly employed as a filler and stretcher of other foods. Also known as carrageen from a village in southwestern Ireland where the seaweed is plentiful, Irish Moss is found clinging to submerged rocks along the shorelines of Canada, New England, the British Isles and Europe as far south as Portugal.

Irish immigrants who found Irish Moss growing on the rugged shores of Canada and New England were the first to gather and use it in America. Irish Moss is harvested throughout the summer months by men in boats who use rakes to gather the 2-foot long stems from among the submerged rocks where they grow.

Hand-gathered Irish Moss, while rare in commerce, is preferred because it is unmixed with other seaweeds. The dried seaweed is soaked in cold water until it swells back to its original bulk. Then it is boiled, turns into jelly as it cools and it is this jelly that serves both medicinal and culinary purposes. It may also be eaten as it is, but is great for thickening soups and stews.

Michigan Autumn

If I could have one wish granted for a city child, it would be to take him/her for a walk along a woods road in Northern Michigan the first week in October. Sometimes I think God gave us autumn so we could fill our eyes and warm our hearts with the glory of color to lighten the bleakness of winter months. If there is one color missing on the hills beside the roads these days, I haven't been able to name it. The first delicate hues of pink and coral flaunting their ethereal loveliness against the stronger tones of orange, scarlet and cinnamon. Blood red maples titillating the dignified green of pines and aspens. Yellow flats of birch tops, like white-clad ladies with Easter bonnets. The mouth-watering hues of shadberry bushes, which seem to have the edge on all the maroons, scarlets and bronzes.

What a privilege to walk through a thicket of color with sunspots picking up bits of magic from the fallen leaves. To round a bend in the road and be confronted with jewel-decked hawthorn trees, their bright berries reminding us of Christmas holly.

Between the gold of witch hazel trees are the delicate yellow blossoms, dainty, beautiful, almost oriental in branch design. If sprayed with clear plastic shellac they will remain whole to delight your eyes all winter. Michigan autumn! There should be a special name for it. But who could coin one comprehensive enough to embrace so much beauty? Citizens of the city, leave your drabness and smog and spend a few days in our colorland, a kaleidoscope of beauty to warm your very soul.

❖

Garlic

To those readers who informed me they loved garlic, and to those whose opinion was anything but enthusiastic regarding that delectable herb, allow me to add a little more information.

We have all read of the boundless treasures found in the tomb of King Tutankhamen, the gold and silver, etc., but no one mentions the fact that there was also many cloves of garlic, proof that it was considered to be of therapeutic value so long ago.

During Caesar's time the Roman army ate large amounts of garlic because they believed it gave them strength and courage in battle. It probably drove the enemy away!

Therapeutically it is considered to be beneficial, for it causes the gastric juices to flow and thus aids in the digestion of food. It also dilates the blood vessels and so is useful in treating high blood pressure.

Few people are aware that there is another type of garlic which is not quite so potent but has the same culinary value. It is the giant garlic. It is much milder than the common garlic and may be used in greater quantities. Chopped finely, it can be added to a salad or, along with parsley may be worked into butter to be used either on crackers and bread, or added to vegetables and scrambled eggs. Chopped coarsely and added to vinegar, it is excellent in making salad dressings and the garlic may be allowed to remain in the vinegar any length of time. I can't imagine cooking a leg of lamb without making slits in the meat and filling them with rosemary and small cloves of garlic. Just be sure to remove the garlic before serving. You may have a guest who says he (she) doesn't like garlic, although they will never know you used it, even though they may marvel at the excellent flavor the lamb.

I'm sorry if I've spoiled your appetite, but you'll never know what you've missed until you try allium sativum.

❖

Seeing Again

Whenever I complain about failing sight, I read a clipping I received from the East a year ago that I'd like to share with you.

"To Bob Edens of South Carolina, yellow is amazing but red is best—although he hasn't seen anything yet he didn't like. He lived 51 years without seeing anything at all, until complicated surgery gave him eyesight. He found it overwhelming.

"I never would have dreamed that yellow was so . . . so yellow. I don't have the words. I'm amazed by yellow. But red is my favorite color. I just can't believe red. Grass is something I had to get used to. I always thought it was just fuzz. But to see each individual green stalk, and to see the hair on my arms growing like trees, and birds flying through the air . . . it's like starting a whole new life. It's the most amazing thing in the world to see things you never thought you'd see.

"I can see the shape of the moon—and I like nothing better than to watch a jet plane flying across the sky leaving a vapor trail. And, of course, sunrises and sunsets. I can't wait to get up each day to see what I can see. I saw some bees the other day and they were magnificent. And I jumped a covey of quail. I had heard quail before, but to see them flying—ah, what an experience!

"I saw a truck drive by in the rain the other day and throw a spray into the air. It was marvelous. And did I mention that I saw a falling leaf, just drifting through the air?" Perhaps we who have sight should be aware of the small, seemingly insignificant things—the beauty of a flower, a mountain, a machine, a sonnet or a symphony.

❖

Morning Gremlins

Everybody has 'em—some more often than others. I knew just what kind of day it was going to be when I turned off the alarm, knocked the electric clock to the floor and broke the strap on my nightgown as I reached for it. I knew, too, when I stepped on the lace at the bottom of said nightgown and almost fell flat on my face in the bathtub. That was when I resolved to abandon flimsy, lace-trimmed, sexy nightwear and stay with the comfort of long-sleeved, untrimmed flannel comfort. Managing to wash my face in cold water and clean my teeth without swallowing the brush, I repaired to the kitchen and breakfast making. How did I know the dog was under my feet? I hadn't yet found my glasses, so his yelp of pain as I trod on him, was justifiably loud.

That morning the gremlins took over the stove. Having been advised by my physician that I must eat more food and start with a good breakfast, I had decided some time ago to have breakfast soon after rising, which is around 6 a.m. and too early to begin anything more important. If your husband believes in a good, substantial breakfast and your tummy suffers from early-morning squeamishness, find yourself a tall, skinny donut dunker. How did I ever put the hash brown potatoes on the high flame, or turn the oven for bacon cooking to 400 when I wanted 300 degrees. And why did those eggs decide to gather brown skirts so fast? Brown was never my favorite color and a brown breakfast day-starter didn't raise my spirits at all. Telephones should never ring early in the morning for me, at least, not when I can knock my hip on a small table holding a plant which impishly scatters soil on the oriental rug. Oh yes! It was my day all right. I knew it even when I sneezed as I was conveying a full cup of hot tea to my lips. I could have gone back to bed, but there will be another day—or will there??

❖

Leeks

What's wrong with leeks? Why do folks turn up their noses when I mention that the leeks in our garden are as big around as a good sized parsnip? These leeks are not to be confused with the wild leek which grows so abundantly in the woods in March and April. "What on earth will you do with them?" I am asked.

Leek (Allium Porrum) is one of the milder members of the onion family, whose natural habitat has been obscured in history. Botanists have been unable to determine its actual native source. Ever since the Welsh soldiers wore leeks in their caps when fighting the Saxons in A. D. 640, the leek has been the symbol of honorable service, and to this day, on the first of March, many a Welshman will wear a boutonniere of fresh leek in honor of David, the patron saint of Wales. It was said that he had once done penance by fasting on leeks only, which he found in the fields.

If you have never heard of Cock-a-leekie, then you don't know a true Scotsman, for that is a dish as popular as Haggis in every Scots household. It is made from chicken, leeks, potatoes, parsley, celery and barley, and it's super!

The Danes, who like their food to not only be well prepared, but to look appetizing too, and one of their leek dishes is as follows. Grontret or Vegetable Castle: 12 large leeks cleaned with the green cut off. Steam until tender. Tie in two bunches and stand upright in center of the dish. Around it in small mounds put cooked brussel sprouts and between the sprouts arrange little dishes with raw shredded carrots which have been mixed with sugar and lemon juice. Serve with melted butter. If that doesn't strike your fancy, leeks au gratin might fill the bill. Two bunches of leeks well washed and trimmed. Cook until tender, about 15 minutes in salted water to cover. Drain and arrange in buttered baking dish. Sprinkle with pepper and cheese and put under broiler until brown. Guess I'll go gather some leeks.

❖

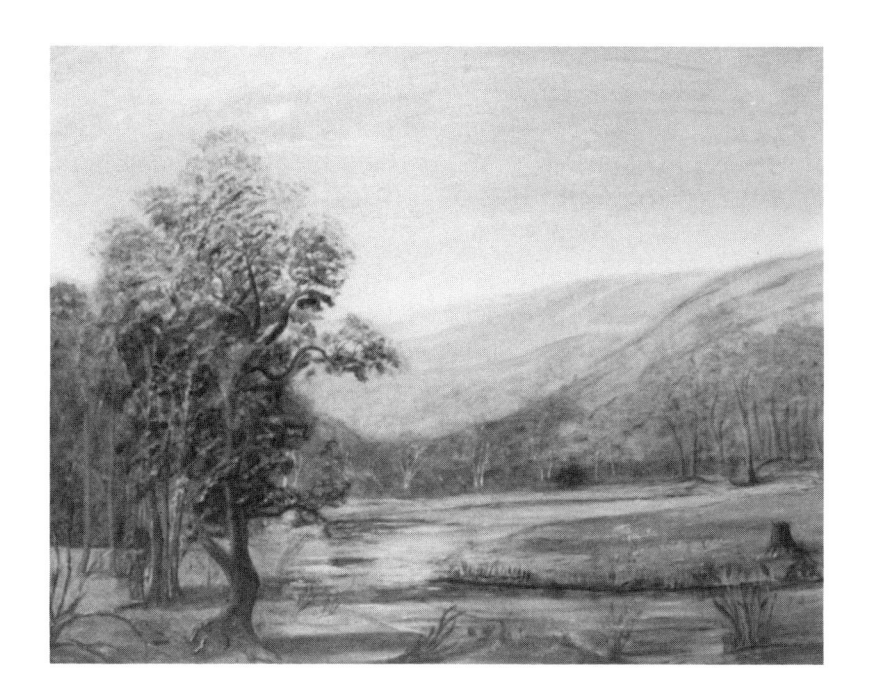

October

If I could choose my favorite month of the year, it would have to be October. It is as capricious as a teenager, and as satisfying as a full-blown love affair.

Our sense of sight is fulfilled by the flamboyant colors of trees as the chlorophyll recedes and the glory of scarlet and gold enlivens the woodlands. Maples, with their brilliant skirts spread out against the dignity of evergreens; shadbush with mouth-watering shades of magenta, deep peach, brilliant orange and the whole gamut of heart-warming vibrancy. October flowers waving a farewell to the roadside weeds. Joe pie, purple asters, yarrow and Queen Anne's lace and the majestic stalks of cattails grace the countryside.

Symmetric V's of migrating geese and the curtains of Northern Lights imbed themselves behind our eyes for winter viewing.

A conservationist wrote, "Almost any writer can describe a beautiful woman, or a baseball game, but William Shakespeare himself could have looked at sumac in early October and hung up his pen."

October! We taste the first honey from the comb, baked apples newly picked from the orchard, the first salmon from the lakes, and roast partridge some friend brought home to you.

Have you felt the pelt of an animal in October, one preparing for outdoor residence during winter? Thick, silky and warm ... or pressed your face against the smoothness of a white birch bark, or run your fingers over the skin of a winter pear?

Smell the earth, giving up its life, but retaining fragrances that cannot be duplicated even by the most renowned "noses" in the perfume-making profession.

Listen to the sound of ducks sailing down the lake, the snort of deer getting ready to mate, the lonesome call of a hoot owl, and the steady lap-lap of running water as it enters the lake.

Someone once referred to October as "the Sabbath of the year."

❖

Myths and Traditions

I have been thinking of the many myths and traditions—magical and religious which have survived almost unaltered right to the present day. For instance, in Crete, the fat, onion-like bulbs of the Sea Squill are hung up by farmers at the entrance to their vineyards to protect the ripening grapes from harmful influences. It is a superstition which seems pointless, but which is explained by tracing the Squill back to the days when it was sacred to the god Pan who protected mortals from evil spirits.

In some parts of Central Europe villagers still plant the succulent House Leek on the roof tiles to prevent their homes from being struck by lightning. The Romans called it Jupiter's Plant because they believed that Jupiter had given it to man to protect his property from being struck by lightning.

Some plants were carried on the person for the benefit of their protective properties. A leaf of Betony carried on the person or in the purse was said to offer protection from witchcraft. A sprig of Mudwort worn inside the shoe was thought to prevent the traveller from becoming tired, an old practice, which surprisingly persisted in East Anglia until the beginning of this century.

These primitive beliefs in the talismanic qualities of plants are, however, by no means confined to the ancient cultures of the world; they abound today in the Third World countries, and you can still be stopped in the heart of London by gypsies hawking sprigs of "lucky heather."

Ah well! I refuse to walk under a ladder and I'm always looking for a four-leaf clover.

❖

My Fig Tree

Yes indeed, plants do have feelings. In fact I believe anything with cell structure is capable of emotion whether it be human, animal or plant life. I have a fig tree in my greenhouse and I love it, but it became infected with rust. One of my gardening books suggested wiping the backs of the leaves with cotton dipped in alcohol. I followed directions, assuring the tree that I was not contributing to its demise as an alcoholic.

Have you ever looked at a man or woman the morning after the night before? That was my fig tree. Droopy, dry, wilted, every leaf curled and dying. Apologizing, I cut off the leaves and fed it a walloping dose of fertilizer. In appreciation, and bearing no malice, it is putting out new leaves.

In late summer I brought indoors a bird of paradise plant and an angel begonia. They were compatible, and grew about the same amount each week. However, the angel begonia suddenly blossomed beautiful pink flowers that overshadowed everything else. What happened was unbelieveable. The bird of paradise closed in upon itself like a pouting child and displayed the most blatant case of jealousy I have ever seen in anything but a human. Yes, I parted them. Madame paradise is now lording it over a group of lowly geraniums, too young to blossom, and she's opening her heart again.

"Throw away your cyclamen and poinsettas when they have finished blooming" says one book on gardening, but I hate disposing of plants as much as I dislike thinning out vegetables in spring. I put a wornout cyclamen and a finished poinsetta under the bench in the greenhouse last May. Those two kids have had fun the last six weeks vieing with each other to see which can grow most in the course of a day or two. I brought them up into the house. The cyclamen is blooming and the poinsetta putting out beautiful leaves.

Can you imagine the cruelty of a man who tells his wife when she bemoans a sick-looking plant, "you probably talked it to death!"

❖

Salt

Have you ever been annoyed when you watched someone add lots of salt to a dinner you have carefully cooked before even tasting the food? Maddening isn't it? I remember as a child reading a story about a chef who killed his master for doing just that. Salt is a necessary ingredient in our diet, but enough is enough and too much can damage our health. When I was young we always bought salt in a block and it was rubbed together to provide salt for the table and for cooking.

There is something almost symbolic about salt and it is certainly essential for man's good health. According to the Bible, salt was considered to be the fitting medium for unalterable exchanges and covenants—a symbol of incorruption and purity. The apostle, speaking of "the salt of the earth" in the book of Matthew, can bestow no greater praise. The devil is said to hate salt because of its purity, and the canny Scotsman is sure that salt will drive away witches.

Salt is indeed the world's finest flavoring, for it brings out the natural flavor of foods. The first written reference to salt is in the book of Job which was written about 300 years before the birth of Christ, and it says "can an unsavory thing be eaten that is not seasoned with salt." Ceasar's soldiers received salt as part of their pay and that is where the word salary originated. It was certainly the chief economic product of the ancient world and many wars were fought for possession of salt sources.

Today, Sodium Chloride, the chemical name for salt, is found in many lakes such as the Great Salt Lake, and in many small inland seas. The waters of the Mediterranean and Caribbean contain the greatest amount of salt among the larger seas. The greatest part of salt used in the United States comes from salt wells in Michigan and Michigan is the largest producer of salt in this country. Is it any wonder we speak of someone we admire as being "the salt of the earth?" It is necessary to use salt frugally and with care.

❖

The Winds

The wind was howling with almost terrifying intensity and the branches of a pine tree beat a sharp tattoo against the sides of the house. The moon was high and the stars were brilliant and I had to leave my bed to watch the night.

Leaves flew hither and yon like small witches flirting with the moon. A high, keening wind echoed from the distant hills, and the air was like nectar. I have heard winds that raced across the fields and made wire fences sing and snap. Winds that picked up the ocean and brought gigantic waves to wash against the sea wall. Winds at sea that whipped against a great liner and sent everyone scuttling for a place to hold on to. Once I heard winds go racing across the hills west of McCormick Lake and it sounded like an express train cutting through the silence of the night. I have seen small whirlwinds that whipped up the earth and carried it in circles way overhead picking up whatever it touched. These were the awesome winds that made my nerves hum and left a trail of fear.

But there are happy winds, light, playful and musical. The soughing sound of wind in tall trees; slim grasses on the sand that leave a pattern where the wind has played with them. There's the wind that comes at sunset after a hot day and makes soft music with the small waves on the lake. I have seen the silky hair of a small child lift like golden strands and have watched a lark wheeling across the heavens, and he sang while the wind produced small nuances of tone.

There are the soft breezes of spring that waft the fragrances of new life to our nostrils and the rustling winds of autumn that stir the dying leaves and shake late fruits from the bushes.

And through it all—I have been so grateful for the gift of hearing.

❖

Chocolate

I like chocolate. During the first World War when I was working in a military hospital and it was impossible to buy chocolate, I made some. Cocoa butter from the pharmacy and nut cocoa and sugar filched from the kitchen when the cook was slightly tipsy and didn't know what I was doing. It wasn't the best chocolate, but every nurse and doctor said it was wonderful. Theobromine is the substance from which chocolate is made and it comes from the cocoa tree, and it has held a place of esteem in the minds of chocoholics for many years. After all, chocolate is said by its lovers to be everything from an aphrodisiac to a cure for loneliness.

In the 1600s, Europeans thought that chocolate not only excited sexual desires but also calmed fevers, cured chronic dyspepsia, and prolonged life. Thomas Jefferson, in the 1700s, spoke of chocolate as being good for health and nourishment. Today, we are sophisticated enough to know that chocolate doesn't calm fevers or prolong life, and it is good to understand that when sugar and fat are added to the bitter cocoa beans it has about 150 calories an ounce. Mixing in small amounts of milk, nuts or fruits doesn't change the calorie content much and only slightly improves the nutritional content.

If a kiss is what you need on a blue day, remember that Hersey makes over 20 million kisses a day, even though scientists tell us that small amounts of a chemical may increase in the brain when cupid's arrow hits. But contrary to rumor, there is no proof that eating chocolate actually creates the euphoria of love—so go easy on the chocolate bars. Chocolate has very little caffeine. You'd have to eat an entire pound of chocolate to get the same amount of caffeine as in one cup of coffee. Nevertheless, chocolate gives many people a lift.

If explorers used it in their climb to the top of Mount Everest and astronauts took it into space, why can't I eat a chocolate bar when my back and legs ache from running around? Isn't it better than a tranquilizer tablet—or a glass of booze?

❖

Autumn's Beauty

Autumn! Month of beauty, when Mother Nature displays her most brilliant assets. Gossamer webs, hanging like pristine scraps of chiffon between wire fences. A time of beautiful sunrises and sunsets. Foliage that fills the memory with music to be enjoyed throughout the months of winter silences.

Summer birds have left after resting quietly for flight discussion on power lines, symmetrically lined up like stones in a necklace. Black squirrels asking whatever happened to summer. There is the friendly chirp of chicadees and the bright plumage of evening grosbeaks to replace the friendly hummingbirds and the cry of the cardinal from a nearby copse.

Today, the sky is a cloth of azure blue with orange-tinged clouds, and the sun-drenched earth was very still. In the woods, lying amongst burnished bracken are the green mosses and the scarlet of wintergreen berries. Rosy apples, like scarlet bouquets hang on the wild, woods trees, an alien spot among the golds, reds and copper of the trees. The last of the mushrooms peek up from the earth. The distant hills across the lake look like the beautiful paisley shawls I remember as a child.

I hear loons across the lake sounding their last "Hurrah" and a "v" of geese wing musically across the asure sky. I wonder what they talk about, and do they carry the hummingbirds under their wings as some folk say? As I walk back towards home, I pass trees still laden with berries. Choke cherries and Pin cherries, fruits which make a wonderful jelly and which wine makers thoroughly enjoy. The fruits of the Hawthorn remind me of the medication this tree now produces.

❖

The "Old Fashioned" Drug Store

As I read about the tragedy of Co-Tylenol, my memory jogged back to my early days in the drug store when Carter's Little Liver Pills, Beechams Pills, Doan's Kidney Pills, yes, even Aspirin tablets were kept safely in drawers that were built into oak fixtures. Even small packages of herbs, which I carried for the convenience of customers who still believed in the healing properties of natural plants, were kept securely away from fingers that could pick up an herb containing a toxic substance when used incorrectly.

Bottles containing such things as Cod Liver Oil, Dr. Hobson's Baby Syrup, S.S.S., Kepler's Malt, Hostetter's Bitters and Lydia Pinkham's Compound were on shelves in glass-covered cases behind the prescription counter or in cases above the drawers (And yes! There was a Lydia Pinkham. Miss Pinkham was a spirited Quaker lady who lived in Lynn, Massachusetts and made a home remedy concocted for female relatives and friends—a mixture of five botanicals suspended in alcohol.)

One advantage to this type of shelving, is the possibility that the pharmacist would wait on the customer, who was then privileged to seek advice—advice which may well have saved him a doctor's or a hospital bill.

If you have ever seen a small child pick up a crayon or a small piece of candy, you can well imagine how easy it would be for him to pocket a potentially dangerous over the counter drug.

Don't scoff at the "old-fashioned" way of doing things for I believe the drug store of the future will resemble the old apothecary shop, and the pharmacist will not be asked to differentiate between Chanel #5 and Intimate perfume, but may devote his time and knowledge to the job for which he spent years of study. We should be grateful for progress but let us not forget that our forebears were well endowed with common sense.

❖

Trees for Health and Food

September—and the trees are already showing their beautiful autumn colors. I wonder how many of us realize the therapeutic value these trees give to the world, both medicinally and as food. Walnut trees, both black and white walnut leaves are boiled to be used as an effective hair dye and the bark is an astringent. The oak tree, which showers so many acorns on us, was used by the Indians to treat consumption, and the kernels of those acorns were a definite cure for diarrhea. Turpentine and gums are also extracted from the bark. Ironwood, those forty foot trees growing on M-32, provide a tea made from the heart of the tree which was used for dyspepsia, neuralgia, and intermittent fevers. The beautiful elm, with its spreading branches was also used for softening hardened tissues and tumors. The soaked leaves were also used to cure leprosy.

One of my old herbal books gives credit to the chestnut tree for providing tea made from the green leaves, a remedy for whooping cough and for diarrhea. And in case you think the magnificent birch is too beautiful to be useful, juice from the young leaves is a specific for kidney and bladder troubles, and the bark is also used in medicine. Balm of Gilead—I still remember buying a bag of the buds of this tree many of which grow in Alpena. The Indians considered the buds of this tree a highly effective medicine. Many years ago I received a prescription for Balm of Gilead buds. I thought my customer had met up with an Indian physician, but he informed me it was for his asthma.

Need I say anything about the magnificent maples? Today they are already wearing garments of scarlet, gold, and russet and they provide us all with the syrup we enjoy on our morning pancakes. We cannot however, forget the sassafras, or the old song "I Got So Thin On Sassafras Tea I Could Hide Behind a Straw." Yes, people did make a tea which slimmed them down from the bark of the sassafras.

"For we can make liquor from walnut tree chips to sweeten our lips." —Thoreau.

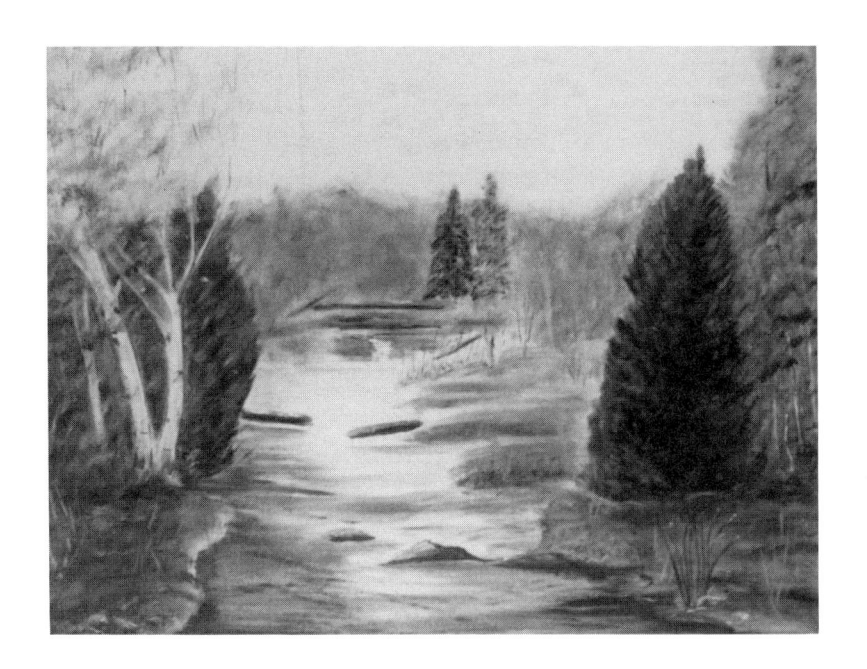

Time for Aloneness

It is October the sixth and what a beautiful world autumn created for us. This morning I watched as the fog slowly lifted to reveal the rhapsody of color across the distant hills. The subtle, artistic blending of greens, gold, crimson and startling yellows that seem to make the woods sing, and form a kaleidoscope of beauty.

Flamboyant crimson of maples, golden yellow birch whose glow enters the house with a brilliance that lights up every corner.

Oh yes! We have our dull days, but I'll take fifty dull days for the sheer pleasure of such a day as this. Clouds that dance across a soft blue sky, and send down reflections into the rippling waters of the lake and streams. The V of large groups of migrating geese, who, I swear, fly a little slower as they pass over the autumn glory.

There is a time when we need to be alone. It is a time to evaluate things. The quality of our life, the things which make for happiness, our values and our deficiencies. To me, the time for aloneness is when the sun has set and the afterglow has receded into the distant hills and the world seems to stand still. Through the veil of darkness, a star twinkles, a bird flutters and small creatures stir the burnished leaves. There's the soft lap-lap of water in the distance and the melancholy lowing of cattle to the north.

The velvet curtains of night obliterate the commercial sounds of day. Feel the presence of those we have loved who have left us, and savor that moment. Believe that we can make a better world. Believe that we are our brother's keeper. "Stand still and know that God is near..."

❖

It Is Autumn

The paisley patterns of gold and red have faded from the landscape and a mystical grey lays a pattern across the distant hills from trees that have lost all leaves. Mist rises from the lake in early morning trying to catch the light from the rising sun. Tall pines, like proud sentinels, stand between the naked branches of oak, maple and birch. Perhaps they are telling us "See, we are still here."

The paths of the woods are alive with the brilliant green of mosses which will remain green even through the first snowfall.

The warm of wintergreen berries peep out from under the glossy leaves, their sharp taste a contrast from the sweetness of blackberries.

The golden, oriental-looking blossoms of witch hazel are brightening the dull woods. I almost feel sorry when I see the open trucks in the eastern states laden with the branches and blossoms of this bush which are being taken to the distillery. But then I remember how often I use the distilled witch hazel for bruises, tired eyes, hemorrhoids, broken blood vessels and so many other ailments. And what would we do without a witch hazel branch as a divining rod for finding water and minerals?

It is autumn. Lianas of mist curl along the shoreline of the lake and ripples are being driven by a north wind.

Birds have found the feeders and are hungrily consuming sunflower seeds. The friendly chickadees and nuthatches watch from nearby branches and the greedy blue jays fill their tummies. A pair of bald eagles fly gracefully across the lake. Are they wondering how much longer fish will be available?

Autumn! The painting fingers of October and early November will soon be gone; the pristine flakes of snow will replace the golden leaves and Mother Nature will be putting on her thinking cap, and wondering what she can send us next.

Witch Hazel

I am patiently waiting to gather my annual bouquet of witch hazel blossoms, bright, oriental in appearance and beautiful. I think witch hazel is one of my favorite remedies for so many small ailments, and it is free for the gathering, but can also be bought in the drug store.

In 1919 I was working in a military hospital in Birmingham, England, when I had a case of conjunctivitis which was completely cured by witch hazel. So, all my life I have depended upon this valuable, natural medication for many ailments. If you have had one of those days when the toast burned, and you put a red sock with the white clothes when you did the laundry and you really feel depressed, soak two pads with witch hazel and put on your eyes. Lie down and think of something lovely. You'll feel completely refreshed and maybe, just maybe, your husband will tell you he really likes pale pink shirts!

Witch hazel is a rather tall bush and the parts used are the leaves, bark and twigs, and those twigs have long been used as divining rods to locate water. The leaves have long been used for bleeding hemorrhoids, also as an enema, and for ulcers and nosebleeds. Also for sprains and bruises and even blood clots. In cases of diarrhea it is used as an enema or by taking 30 grains of the dried leaves internally.

The constituents of this herb are tannic and gallic acids, a small amount of volatile oil and an unknown bitter principle. I hope that some day that bitter principle will be identified and prove to be an invaluable drug. Most women know the value of witch hazel as a skin freshener and it is a safe treatment for skin blemishes. The Indians poured hot water over the leaves of the plant and applied them as hot as possible to swellings, bruises and sprains. It is excellent for minor burns and scalds, and if a wet cloth is applied to a burst vein, the bleeding will be arrested until medical help is reached.

Bald Eagles

Early Autumn . . . the time of beautiful sunrises and glorious sunsets! Foliage that fills the memory with music to be enjoyed through the months of Winter whiteness. Summer birds have left us and the friendly chirp of chickadees, the brilliant plumage of evening grosbeaks and the blue of the jays has taken over to bring joy to our bird feeders.

Yesterday the sky was a cloth of azure blue with orange-tinged clouds, and the sun-drenched earth was very still. Like dancers vying for supremacy in a ballet, three huge bald eagles sailed majestically across the sky under the dome of cobalt. I wondered how they managed to maintain that smooth glide with barely a movement of wings—just back and forth with such graceful symmetry I began to think they might be three jets practicing formation flying.

They disappeared across the lake until they appeared to be no bigger than sparrows, then, when I had bid them farewell they suddenly appeared again. Perhaps they were looking for food, or for some small animal, but all their attention seemed focused on that beautiful display of graceful flight. They were majestic, with their white heads and graceful forms adding dignity to their flight.

Their nests are up the river, and although they are supposed to migrate during the Winter, I have seen many a bald eagle during those cold months. As I watched them today, I remembered the words of Mr. Burroughs, who so beautifully expressed his thoughts of the bald eagle:

"He draws great lines across the sky; he sees the forests like a carpet beneath him; he sees the hills and valleys as folds and wrinkles in a many-colored tapestry; he sees the river as a silver belt connecting remote horizons. We climb mountain peaks to get a glimpse of the spectacle that is hourly spread beneath him. Dignity, elevation, repose are his. I would have my thoughts take as wide a sweep. I would be as far removed from the petty cares and turmoils of this noisy and blustering world."

❖

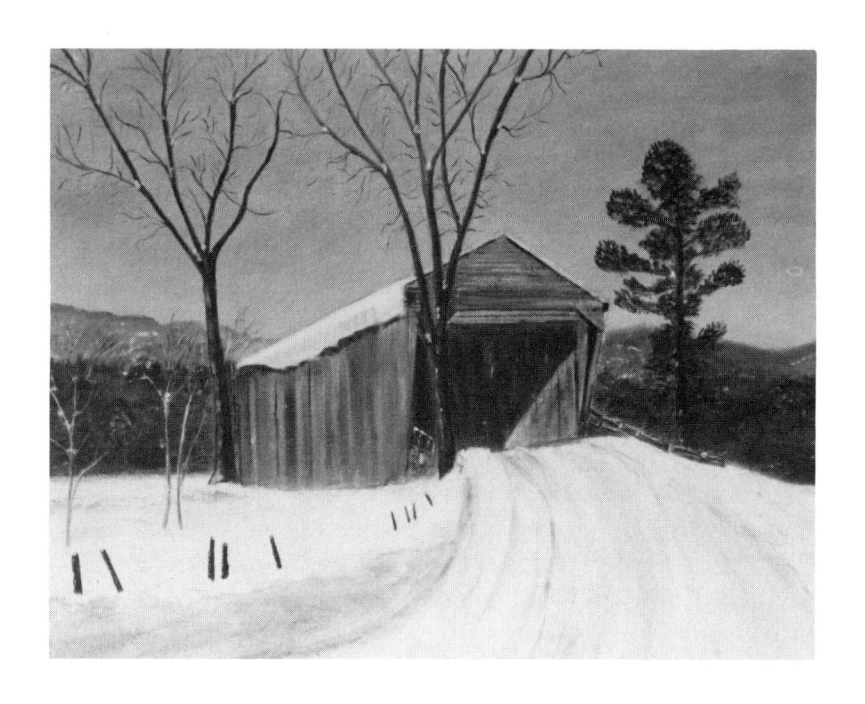

Our Beautiful World

I have just returned from a trip through New England and my eyes have absorbed enough color to warm my heart all winter. Hedgerows, thick with the light mahogany of sumac laced with orange-fruited bittersweet. In New Hampshire, roses were blooming on trellises in front of immaculate white houses, absorbing the fall sunshine, and along the paths at the edge of beaches. Rosehips, like ruby jewels, were large, ripe and ready for picking.

Waving beach grasses with their warm, toasty fragrance made me think of winter bouquets. Gardens were alive with marigolds, yellow, gold and scarlet, interspersed with nasturtiums in many brilliant colors.

Clumps of evergreens clipped into geometrical shapes, reminded me of the old Victorian gardens in England and I recalled the scolding I once had from a gardener when I ran my hand across the top of a juniper that had been shaped to resemble a harp.

Across the hills, the tips of maples rose like flames against the dark evergreens, and birches were wearing their cloths of autumn gold. I stood on a knoll and watched the Atlantic ocean, its waves lapping gently against the sea wall as the tide rolled in, but I remembered how turbulent that ocean could be at times, and I thought that is how life could be. Peaceful 'tis true, but peacefulness has to be shattered at times, how else would we appreciate tranquility. But, perhaps my main thoughts were, "What a beautiful world we have."

❖

Autumn Tapestries

Rumble! Flash! The rush of wind and the sound of thunder and the heavenly fragrance of rain on the warm earth. The pungent smell of burning wood in the early-morning chill. Flocks of small birds laced like jewels of jet along the telephone wires. Tall grasses waving along the roadside and maple trees flaunting crimson bits of leaves along the branch tips. It all adds up to late summer. The St. John's Wort with golden blossoms and bronze tansey heads and lavender joe pye weed ask to be gathered for winter bouquets. The froth of milkweed blossoms if getting ready to fly and witch hazel, with its oriental looking blossoms is beginning to ripen. Watercress has dropped its summer bloom and is offering tender green leaves for salad, sandwiches, and that most wonderful of all soups—watercress!

There are a few wild apples the late frost didn't touch; here and there a small quantity of black berries, but choke and pin cherries are ready for picking—wine, jelly, or just canning the juice for a good vitamin-laden winter beverage.

Michigan is the home of the cherry growers and here is a fruit we should use as much as possible, for what is better than a cherry pie when the snow is six feet deep and you are dreaming of spring? How we savor those last few days of summer. Burnished bracken, exotic mosses with wintergreen berries, like ruby jewels, decorating the green.

The lamenting cry of the loons at daybreak. The single note of a bird far back in the woods, like the farewell of a good friend. They come and go, these seasons with their own particular beauty. *"What is beauty never dies but passes into other loveliness."* —Aldrich.

And so, this summer of beauty we have so much enjoyed will pass into the autumn tapestries of color and fragrance, and again we will embrace with joy another season.

❖

A New Day

As I watched the new day opening its arms this morning, the sun came up with brilliant flames of orange and scarlet cutting through the mists of dawn to bathe the woods on the west side of the lake, clothing them in a mantle of magenta. It resembled the foundation an artist might have painted on his canvas before painting a huge mural. The branch of every tree was laced with icy snow, hanging like necklaces from tree to tree, and, as the sun caught them, diamonds sparkled and a new day was born. A black squirrel appears, blinking his eyes at the unexpected brilliance of dawn light, and headed for breakfast at the bird feeder.

Winter wonderland! Incomparable beauty! As the sun rose, the green of the trees on the distant hills appeared, with the cap of the hills covered with hoar frost like a pale pink frill on a lady's mantle, and the jet black of an eagle flew across the landscape as if to show his ownership this beautiful morning.

Noonday was a palace of crystal, the white of birches cutting through the snow-laden evergreens. Sharp, snapping sounds, like snapping whips came heavily from laden branches anxious to unload their burden of ice. Chickadees twittered thanks for their well-stocked feeder, while blue jays fought over a piece of stale bread and evening grosbeaks took advantage of the fracas to clean up the sunflower seeds. Listen to the silence. Hum a melody. Breathe the pure oxygen. This is your world, to berate or to enjoy.

Twilight comes in on kitten feet and day ends, like the closing of a good book. Night falls swiftly. The velvety indigo blue of the heavens a perfect foil for the full moon and the adjacent stars. A plane hums across the horizon. A night bird gives a plaintive call, and in the distance a dog barks joyfully.

Surely I hear a voice saying "Be still and know that I am God."

Dr. Diet, Dr. Quiet and Dr. Merryman

Mai Thomas, a delightful writer, found exercise books filled with the old folk remedies of her grandmother, who died at the ripe old age of 95. This delightful character believed in folk lore remedies that had been handed down from mother to daughter. That they were effective is a fact frankly admitted even by members of the medical profession. Here are a few of the items I have read:

"The best physicians are Dr. Diet, Dr. Quiet and Dr. Merryman.

"The surest way to health, say what they will, is never to suppose we shall be ill.

"Most of those evils we poor mortals know, from doctors and imagination flow."

Here are a few of her remedies:

"If you have piles, eat a large, boiled leek.

"If your breath smells strong after onion eating, a cup of strong coffee will remove all smell of onions from your breath.

"A cup of hot water before meals will prevent nausea.

"To make an ant trap, soak a sponge in water and wring it nearly dry. Sprinkle with sugar and lay on a plate by the ants' haunts. As soon as it is full, plunge it into boiling water.

" If slugs are in your garden, put cabbage leaves in the oven until soft, rub with drippings and lay wherever the slugs are. The leaves will soon be covered with slugs and snails.

" For hiccup, dip a piece of sugar in vinegar and eat it slowly. Or, moisten brown sugar with vinegar and take a teaspoonful. The effect is almost instantaneous.

" For sunburn, wash the face with sage tea.

"Should warts be bothering you, rub them daily with radish, or with the juice of marigold flowers. It seldom fails. Rubbing the wart with a piece of raw meat is also good.

"Dandelion leaves are very good for the heart and liver and are delicious when added to salads.

"Parsley tea stimulates the kidneys and is good for rheumatism. Drink plenty of it before meals.

"If you have corns, apply bruised ivy leaves. In two weeks they will drop out."

So, there are a few tips from a wise old lady!

❖

Six Herb Vinegar

I have just finished making what I call Six Herb and Garlic Vinegar. Combine sweet basil, summer savory, tarragon, oregano, lemon balm and sweet margoram. Bring to a simmer for about five minutes. Strain, cool and put into sterile bottles. Add one clove of garlic and freshly gathered herbs. This is excellent when making salad dressings and the older it is the better it tastes. These end-of-the-season gatherings are always interesting.

Don't forget the rosehip marmalade. When the seeds of the fruit have been removed the pulp may be put through the blender to reduce the bulk readily. Add a little lemon juice to both the jam and the jelly. If chokecherries are abundant in your woods try making chokecherry brandy. (This is not intended for teetotalers.)

Strip the wild berries from the stems, crush and boil with a cup of water to a quart of juice for at least half an hour. Strain through a jelly bag and mix with a quart of sugar to a pint of juice. One pint of this juice is then added to a quart of commercial brandy—Happy Holidays!

Do try to use the bright, red heads of the scarlet sumac. Bruise the fruit with a potato masher in water. Strain through a fine cloth to remove all the hairs. Sugar and ice may be added for taste. This drink will resemble a pink lemonade and provide a slightly acid, flavorful drink. Why not dry a few of the berries for a good winter drink. The vitamin C content is abundant.

Take advantage of the things that are free and are good for us. Remember that rosehips contain 24 times the vitamin C of oranges. If the Scandinavian people can use rosehips for use in soups, for sprinkling over cereals and for making hot and cold drinks—why not us?

❖

Wild Foods

Delicious wild foods grow everywhere. For example, there is the familiar berry that, although you maybe never sampled it, has the flavor of fresh applies. Moreover, its juice is from 6 to 24 times richer in Vitamin C than even orange juice. Throughout much of the country, you can pick all you want the greater part of the year, even when temperatures fall below zero as low as 60 degrees. It is easy to recognize this fruit, and anyone with the least knowledge of the outdoors will not gather the wrong berry by mistake. It is the rose hip, the ordinary seed pod of roses everywhere.

Perhaps you know all there is to know about rose hips, but it is worth renewing the information. There are at least 35 different species of wild roses growing along the roadsides, fences and streams in the United States. The hips, or haws as we sometimes call them, are round and smooth and grow from fragrant flowers, usually pink or red. These fruits will remain on the bush throughout winter and well into spring.

They are delightful to eat either raw, dried and made into juice, jam or jelly. They are strong medicine to boot. Studies in Idaho found the scurvy-preventing vitamin in the raw pulp, running from 4,000 to nearly 7,000 per pound. Daily human requirements, estimated to be 60 to 75 milligrams, provide a yardstick for this abundance. These rose hips, the experts say, have as much vitamin C as an orange.

We don't pay as much attention to these gratuitous vitamins in the United States and Canada, but in England, in World War II, some five million pounds of rose hips were gathered from the roadside and put up to replace the then-scarce citrus fruits. Dried and powdered, rose hips are sold in Scandinavian countries for use in soups, for mixing with milk or water to make hot and cold drinks, for sprinkling over cereals, etc. all of which they do admirably.

"And God said, 'Behold, I have given you every herb bearing seed, which is upon the face of the earth.'"

❖

Elderberry

The fruit-bearing trees and bushes are beginning to bring in their harvest, although I saw some flowers on an elderberry bush a few days ago, and I thought about the wonderful elderberry blow my Granny used to make. The medicinal uses of the elderberry have long been known; in fact, an ointment for healing the sores on animals is made from the blossoms, and a similar ointment is recommended to beautify the complexion. I don't remember the exact formula, but I do know the blossoms were steeped in lard for an hour and then strained.

My first recollection of elder was what, in those days, we called elder blow. Today they might be named elderflower waffles. Wash a bunch of the blossoms, shake well, dip in waffle batter and fry in deep fat. The frying is but a minute or two after which the waffle is put on paper towel to drain, dipped in fine sugar, and—well, just try them.

Perhaps the most well-known use for elderberries is the wine. A beautiful pale yellow wine of delicate flavor can be made from the blossoms. To one quart of the stemmed elderflowers, add three gallons of water, five pounds of sugar and ferment this mixture with yeast. After standing nine days, strain and add three pounds of raisins. This should be stored in a cool dark place in an oak keg for six months, then carefully bottled.

If pie is your 'thing,' do make an elderberry pie. Cook five cups of fully ripe elderberries in half a cup of cold water over a very slow fire, first adding the juice and grated rind of one lemon. Now add $1\ 1/2$ cups of sugar and one scant tablespoon of cornstarch. Stir until the mixture begins to thicken. Pour into unbaked pie shell and bake in a hot oven.

Do remember that this wild fruit is exceedingly rich in calcium, vitamin A, iron and potassium.

❖

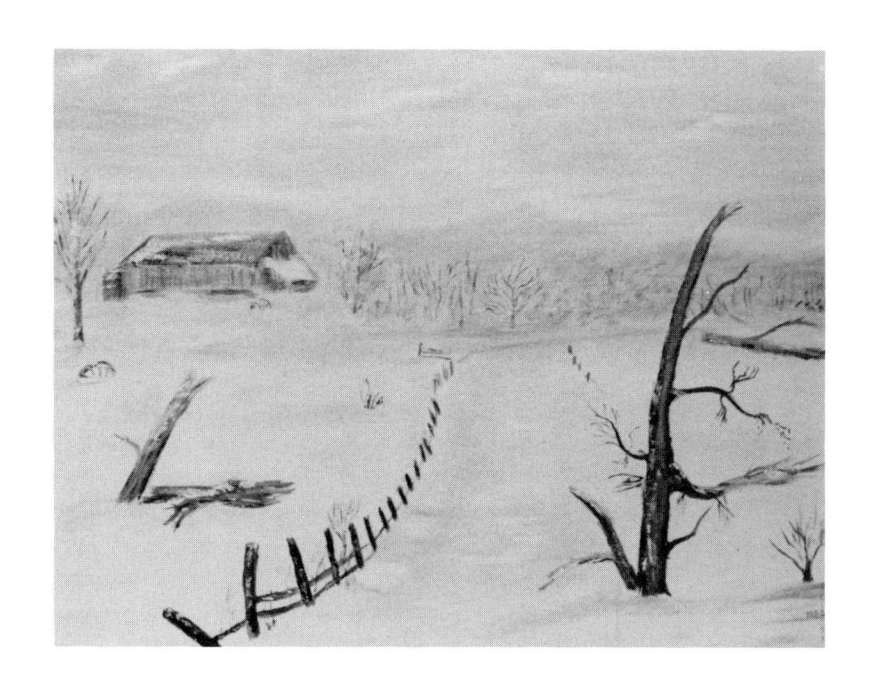

Winter Stillness

There's a pristine beauty over the whole countryside this morning. It is as if Mother Nature recognized the holiness of this season and wished to participate. The sun rose with hauteur frostiness, but as it touched the hills it changed to a rosy, warm pink. Frost had preceded dawn light and awaited the sun to turn the magic of hoar frost into fairyland. Mist rolled in gently from the river and ushered the air with its frost into the pine trees and suddenly green was glory. Sunrise picked up the patterns on the ice of the lake, geometrical, fanciful, abstract—designs created by the wind, ice and snow.

There is a path that zigzags the width of the lake and I wonder if a leprechaun with a giant broom tried to make a path for the deer to cross, or perhaps he was interested in the otter frolicking at the end of the river.

Sunrise has brought in clouds, tinged with orange and framed with the blue-gray of snow clouds. With a joyful flutter of wings, evening grosbeak, blue jays and chickadees, like a cloud of softness, dart across the sky to settle on the feeders for breakfast. They wait respectfully and perhaps a little resentfully for the squirrels who had arrived earlier. There's a peace, a quietness, a stillness that soothes the spirit and prepares us for another day. The crackle of ice, the call of a bird, soft winds that sigh in the tall pines like sorrowing spirits. Across the lake, in the hills, hoar frost appears like pink frosting on a birthday cake for a beloved friend.

Another morning. Another day, and somehow, through the stillness of early morning, a voice saying with reverence, "May you have a happy and peaceful Christmas."

❖

My Music

I turned on the radio very early this morning, and someone was playing an old Scotch ballad that took my memory way back along the years, to when I sat and listened to my mother and dad as they sat before the fire in the evening. My mother played her Irish harp and dad sang his songs in a beautiful tenor voice. They both died when I was very young, but that melody survives in my heart.

Music!! Of course it hath charms! Is any sound more satisfying than the sound of a choir or a congregation singing those grand old hymns? In a small chapel or under the roof of a great cathedral, they touch the very heart.

During World War I, three members of the hospital staff of the hospital in which I worked in England were given a well-earned morning off duty. We spent the time breakfasting in a beautiful old inn in Malvern Hill. After breakfast we climbed through the mist to the top of the hill, and as we stood in the sunlight, a group of soldiers on R & R at the inn began to sing "It's a Long, Long Way to Tipperary." Never have I heard such longing in men's voices. I prayed they might live long enough to go back to their Tipperary and to this day I hear those voices when someone plays the ballad.

I've been repairing a scarf which I first wore when I went to the opera to hear and see *Madame Butterfly*, and with every stitch I hear the beautiful arias of longing and loving. Do you remember your first date and the first dance? Can you hear the music today without remembering how you worried your partner might not like you? I used to sing a lullaby to my young daughter. The lyrics were my own, but not until years later did I remember it was a melody my Irish granny hummed as she kneaded her bread.

Music! Can it influence your life? Is a tranquilizer what you need, or should the sound of an old ballad soothe your spirits, or a slow waltz remind you of a beautiful evening with a loved one. Have you ever really analyzed the effect of long lost melodies upon our peace of mind and happiness?

"The man that hath no music in himself is fit for treason," says Shakespeare.

———— ❖ ————

Plants' Feelings

Yes! I do talk to my plants, and *no*, they don't answer me. And to those of my friends who think I am a nut, I am when it comes to plants and flowers.

Plants, like children, respond to a light slapping as I recently proved when I gave a cactus the back of my hand. It hadn't bloomed since Christmas of 1990, just sat there looking rather ugly, so I chastened it! Today it is full of buds and will soon be a blooming mass of blossoms. I did, however, drizzle a spoonful of castor oil over the soil which might have loosened things up a bit.

I think communication is possible among all forms of cellular life, so why not plants. All winter the large bay window is full of plants. They all thrive. Blossoms are abundant. They are happy and when it is time to move them to a less sunny place, they pout! A large Boston fern became quite belligerent, dropped its leaves and turned brown. I started giving it some of my morning tea and it quickly responded to kindness, so much so I feed it a drop of tea each morning.

Some time ago, I took a cutting from a beautiful Kalancoe and she stopped blooming. The cutting grew and was soon covered with beautiful blossoms. I put it next to the mother plant and admonished "look what your child can do." Jealousy? Rivalry? Who knows, the mother plant is blooming as she never bloomed before.

What about incompatibilities? If humans find people with whom they cannot get along, why not plants? An impatience hates a Boston fern. My bird of paradise plant would rather die than sit next to a cactus, and that is what it almost did! There are several plants that react violently to a wandering Jew and the African violet prefers to live with its own kind.

Do plants have feelings? Why not ask them?

❖

Sesame Seeds

When a delightful lady confessed that she thought she might become addicted to sesame seeds, I was tempted to tell her that maybe in a previous life she might have been an Oriental lass living in the days of the Arabian Nights, for this annual herb was first grown in China and Turkey and of course, other parts of the Orient. Today it is also grown in the southern part of the United States where the seeds are expressed for the oil we use in salad dressings.

Sesame seed is one of the oldest spices known to mankind. There is an ancient legend with writings dating back to 2,300 B. C. revealing that legendary Assyrian gods drank sesame seed wine while creating the earth. More than four billion pounds of sesame seed is grown annually throughout the world. Perhaps it is not as popular in this country as it is in the Orient, but in the last few years more cooks are learning to use this nutty flavored seed in their cooking.

In the Near East a confection called Halvah is made from the seeds and this is the popular confection of these people. We use them in bread, rolls, cookies and in many other dishes which call for a topping of breadcrumbs, for the almost nut flavor adds greatly to many foods.

Sesame seeds are extremely nutritious for they contain calcium and Vitamin C in large amounts. Lecithin, B12 and Vitamin D are also present in surprising quantity.

The seed was first brought to South America by slaves who called it "benne" seed an African name which is still used in many parts of the South.

These seeds are great when combined with cheeses. Serve with butter over noodles and vegetables and create a new taste treat for your family. Here is a recipe I think you will like. I call them Benne Wafers: $3/4$ cup melted butter, $1\ 1/2$ cups firmly packed brown sugar, 1 teaspoonful vanilla, 1 egg, 1 cup toasted sesame seed (toast in skillet in a little butter), $1\ 1/2$ cups sifted flour, $1/4$ teaspoon baking powder, $1/4$ teaspoonful salt.

Cream butter and sugar. Add vanilla and egg and beat till light. Stir in seeds, baking powder, flour and salt. Drop by $1/2$ teaspoonful onto a well greased pan; allow for spreading. Bake at 375 for ten minutes and remove from pan at once.

If you don't use sesame seeds you are really losing a terrific nutritive food.

❖

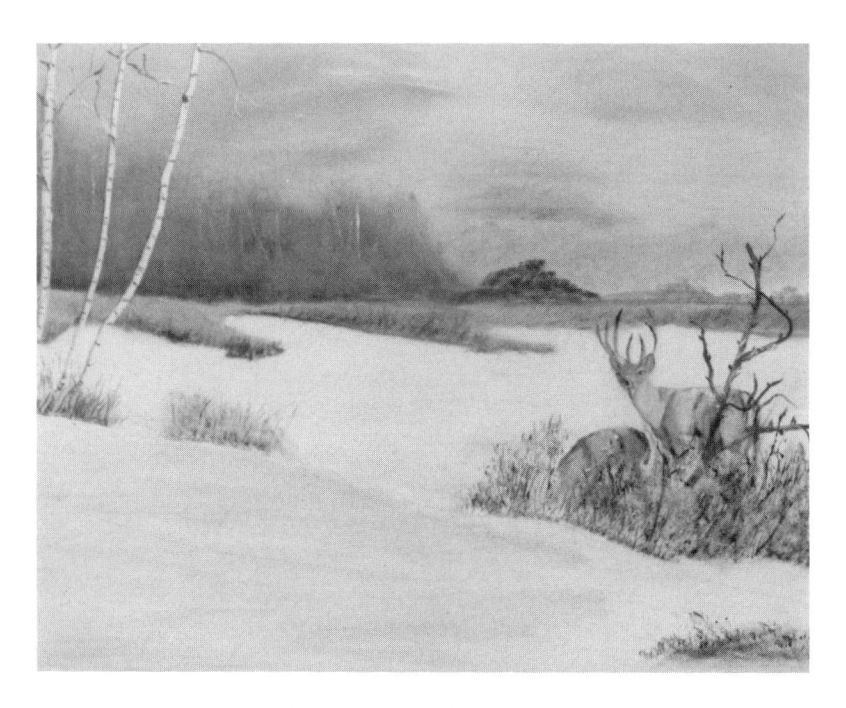

Beauty of Winter

Despite the wind, ice and sub-zero temperatures, there's something in the beauty of winter days that is very special. The rising sun bathing the western hills with a warm, rosy glow, scintillating bits of ice like daytime glow worms on the pristine whiteness of the trees, and the whipping winds lifting the snow from the lake, carrying it heavenwards like the smoke from a witch's fire. Where else, but in this winter wonderland can one see the geometric magic of the patterns fashioned by frost, or a row of spruce trees clad in white like ladies-in-waiting.

This morning I saw some evening grosbeaks sitting in a small maple and looking like ripe, yellow fruit, wondering which bird feeder had the best seed.

The deer walk slowly and delicately across the lake, after long contemplating whether or not there was peril in crossing. Hunger always wins. A pair of otters cavort in the water of the stream that enters the lake—at least I presume they are otters. Occasionally there's a slight argument about the possession of a fish. Squirrels compete gymnastically to reach bird food suspended on a line above the porch, and occasionally there's a raucous cry of a blue jay who feels left out of things.

Let your eyes follow the sun as it penetrates the grey mist of a dull morning. It plays hide and seek across the distant hills and makes me think of the many nuances of good music with its light and shade. Ah yes! The days are short and snow lies heavy upon the land, hiding the debris that careless hands have cast aside. But can spring be too far away? If there were no winter, what would happen to the joy of watching the earth come to life beneath the comforting cover of snow. I want to watch the trailing Arbutus unfold its blossoms; see the various shades of hepatica; hear the song of the first robin, and rejoice that I am alive to enjoy it all.

—— ❖ ——

Aloe Vera

Although I have written about aloe before, I have recently received from *Tribune* readers a request to repeat the story of this precious plant.

Down through the ages, primeval healing practices involved the use of this amazing tropical plant which is grown in South Florida and other tropical regions. It is mentioned in the Bible and throughout ancient history. Recent research into ancient history has disclosed the fact that our early Egyptian civilization used aloe for beautifying and preserving skin. I didn't know that it would also reduce wrinkles, but if you see me wearing an aloe face mask, you'll know what I'm up to.

In case you have ever wondered what was the beauty secret of Cleopatra, wonder no more; for it is believed that Cleo knew all about aloe and used it while the rest of the women of her day wondered what was her secret.

Today, aloe is used by physicians for burns, internal and external ulcers, ringworm, insect bites and many people with nervous stomachs find that chewing a piece of the bottom of an aloe leaf will give relief. We are now told that the juice from the aloe is used in radiation burns.

Care must be taken when pulling a leaf from the plant, for the yellow juice which is in the lower part of the leaf next to the main stem is in the aloin which has been used in medicine as a laxative for many years.

It is the *clear gel* which contains the miracle healing properties. This gel will positively regenerate skin tissue, heal and restore damaged flesh. It is interesting to note that research has shown that the crystal clear gel from the aloe is, in itself, bacteriostatic.

I have had reports from people who tell me that aloe has given them relief from pain both topically and below the skin, and they also tell of getting relief from arthritis, ulcers, indigestion, constipation and many other ills.

The pure gel may be bought in tubes and 12 ounce bottles. It contains no other ingredient and I have personally found it to be invaluable.

Guess I'll give my wrinkles a dose right now.

— ❖ —

Aloneness Is Needed

I swear there was almost a look of pity in the eyes of a friend when I told her my husband and I would be alone for Christmas. A good fire, conversation, fine music and memories to lace the silences—those silences so necessary for a healthy outlook on life. Should one feel regret for having such a day to tuck into the book of one's life? Aloneness and loneliness. What a difference there is in the meaning of the two words. Aloneness is something we all need if we are to maintain our sanity. It's a time to evaluate ourselves and our worth. A time to listen to the inner feelings and to recuperate from the pressures of everyday living.

The next few weeks of winter will afford us many days of aloneness. Perhaps we should take advantage of this time and regard it as an opportunity to become acquainted with ourselves, and, if we are fortunate, to have loved ones near with whom to share our ideas. There are people who shun solitude and need to be with other people all the time. They are running away from life and missing one of the greatest privileges—companionship with oneself.

Life is demanding. No longer do we have the simple things of yesteryear when just plain existence depended upon our own ingenuity; when we didn't have time to wonder what we could do with our spare hours. There were no spare hours. Each moment was a time of giving—giving of ourselves and our efforts. But because chores were often done alone, there was also the opportunity to look inwards at ourselves; to ask questions; solve problems, and somehow maintain a serenity alien to many people today.

Thoam De Quincey wrote these words: "Solitude, though it may be silent as light, is like light, the mightiest of agencies: for solitude is essential to man."

❖

Crystallized Flowers

I often decorate a dessert with crystallized flowers or mint leaves. They are interesting and edible and some of my friends have asked for the recipe, so I'll share it. I took it from an old English book which I received when I was eight years old for, of all things, constant attendance at Sunday School!

If you are fortunate enough to have the fragrant parma violets in your garden, use them for they are best, Red rose petals are most colorful for crystalizing. Any kind of mint leaves, either apple, orange, spearmint or plain lamb mint will do. These are particularly effective on a lemon gelatin salad or tossed into a fruit salad. Even small nasturtium leaves are good on a molded vegetable salad. Try them all; you will be interested.

Any blossom can be crystallized. It is better, however, to use the flowers you know are edible. Gather the blossoms after a dry spell when there is no possibility of dew being left on them.

Dip them into very thin royal icing made from white of an egg well whisked to a stiff froth and sufficient icing sugar to mix. It should be thin enough to drain off easily.

Color it or flavor it if you wish with rose water, violet essence etc. I don't use anything. It really isn't necessary.

Place the dipped and well-coated petals on a wire rack, and before the icing sets, sprinkle with castor sugar (this is regular sugar). Allow them to dry in a cool oven with the door open. I use a temperature of about 150 degrees. Store in airtight tin. When making mint leaves use one drop of *pure* peppermint. This adds to the flavor and is good. Try putting mint leaves in a fruit salad, or decorate a vegetable gelatin salad with them. Anything that adds a little charm, or originality to food is worthwhile.

❖

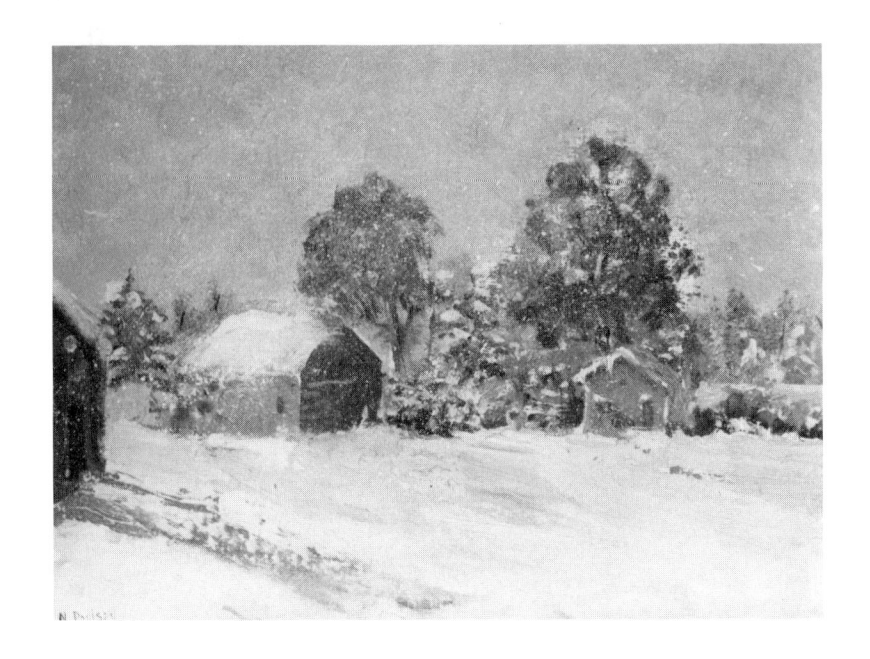

Hoarfrost

It had been a bitterly cold night. The wind had whistled around the chimney with weird sounds, and there wasn't a star to be seen in the darkness of the sky. Then I heard the freezing rain. Morning came all too soon, for who wished to be greeted by darkness and an icy glare? It was dark when I sat before the front window overlooking the lake—sad and depressing. What kind of day lay ahead? I drank my morning tea slowly and repeated my usual morning prayer.

It was then that something wonderful happened. The first rays of sunlight rose from the eastern horizon and caught the top of the hills in the north across the lake and the day came alive. A hoarfrost covered the trees and, as the first rays of sunshine bathed the treetops, they were suddenly a pastel pink and later they deepened to a light red.

Why did I think that amongst the gloomy days of life there is always something beautiful? Later in the morning I made a trip to town, driving slowly and feasting my eyes—and yes—my heart on the frost-covered bushes glistening in the sunlight. A few deer crossed the road and I am sure they enjoyed the brilliance of trees they could feast on. A huge bird flew through the treetops, sending a shower of icy particles to the ground. What a world! We don't have 70 degree temperatures, but in our north country of Michigan, we have beauty, natural beauty, enjoyed by birds, animals and humans.

The eagles seem to have decided to stay with us this winter and two adults wing their way across the lake many times a day. Blue jays, woodpeckers, and many small birds wait patiently in nearby bushes. May we always have the strength to face the darkness, and life enough to look for the beauty.

❖

Hobbies

Yesterday, I received a letter from a friend thanking me for getting her interested in the hobby of painting. Why do people complain that they are bored? I cannot put out any empathy when I talk with these people. Perhaps because I can't remember ever being bored. If spare time is the boring period, why not take up a hobby. I'll guarantee boredom will soon be in the used-to-be bracket. A hobby can be almost anything a person likes to do in his/her spare time. People take up hobbies because they bring happiness, friendships, knowledge and relaxaton, and sometimes even wealth. They make life easier and provide a good balance between work and play for those people who work hard and have many responsibilities.

An outdoor hobby is a change from indoor work. A house painter might like to paint pictures. An editor may enjoy writing poetry. It is a matter of individual taste and no one can tell you what to choose. Doctors have found hobbies of great help with patients recovering from mental and physical illnesses. Many veterans have recovered the use of their hands, arms or legs, by following a hobby. Many hobbies which were taken up as a pastime, have ended as lifetime jobs of importance. Hobbies have also led to some of the world's greatest inventions and discoveries. Many persons enjoy hobbies that require action, such as tennis, baseball, basketball, etc.

Since primitive times men have enjoyed tests of their strength and endurance. There are people who prefer to make things with their hands, many kinds of tools and materials, wood, brass, iron, plastics, glass, etc. Think of the men who had hobbies that have given great pleasure to the world.

The new year is upon us. Don't complain about being bored. With a hobby, you will not only be helping yourself, but others also.

Do please remember you can obtain books from your library on almost any subject you choose to study. Happy New Year.

❖

Beauty Is Everywhere

On Friday, February 4th, the sun came up with an unusual brilliance as though telling us mortals the world could still be beautiful. Every twig was covered with ice scintillating like diamond pendants from the boughs of the trees. Sunshine shed its brilliance along the hilltops across the lake, and the hoar-frosted trees became pastel shades of pink and lavender, like the frosting on a cake. It was a day to drive through the woods; to stop and admire the unusual beauty of a winter wonderland. Many times I stopped the car and walked into the woods to touch a particular bit of brilliance which I felt was too beautiful to be made of frozen rain, and, as I stood looking up to the globules of irridescence the sun melted a small piece of ice which rolled slowly down the bark, like the tears of the very aged.

And than I heard the song of the Nymphs, sharp, crackling notes of merriment; then silence and a melancholy snip, snap, as small twigs broke under the weight of ice. I tried to think of words I might use to enhance those snapping notes of glee, but the beauty, the pristine purity of the whole world had an aura of holiness—not to be disturbed by lacing the melody with words. It was as if God said, "Stand and listen, and fill your heart with peace."

When the day was over and the sun reluctantly sank into another part of the world, the beauty, reluctant to leave, was etched across the western hills. The tips of evergreens, catching the last rays of sunlight, pointed heavenwards like blades of silver tipped with rose. And then the sun was gone below the horizon.

"What is lovely never dies but passes into other loveliness."

❖

The Power of a Smile

"A soft answer turneth away wrath." That, I'll agree, is true, but how often do we give thought to the tone of voice we use? Last week, a dreary looking clerk bade me "Have a nice day." I should have smiled and thanked her, but I felt as if I had just been sentenced to a life of loneliness. I didn't smile. I felt sad, almost apprehensive. A pickup was what I needed. My memory went back to a day long ago when I went into a small cafe for a cup of coffee and a sandwich. The waitress who served me wished me "Good morning" and her smile was bright, her voice cheerful, and her dark Italian eyes were alight with friendship. Everything that had been worrying me all morning just vanished. It was the joie de vivre in that young woman's voice which quickened the cockles of my heart and made the day joyful again.

There's so much power in a smile. In fact, it's one of our greatest assets. I wonder why we don't use it more, and adopt a cheerful voice to go with it. Even a reprimand given in the right tone of voice loses some of its sting and is far more effective than an abrasive tone. I have a friend who, when I am particularly vocal, looks me in the eyes and says "faker." Does it hurt? No, because the tone of voice is laced with a bit of love.

I always answer the phone with a "Good morning" or whatever time of day it is. It was many years ago when I became acutely aware of the importance of *tonal* happiness. Early one morning in the pharmacy, I answered the phone with my usual greeting, "Thank you, I needed a little cheer," was my caller's greeting. It was many days later when I heard that my caller had spent a discouraging night in the hospital with a sick husband.

A smile. A cheerful voice. Just one small candle in a troubled world. Isn't it worthwhile?

❖

"All Is Well"

Living in solitude, I have been privileged to observe many hitherto unnoticed things. I am fortunately situated in my home, for I am high on a hill overlooking McCormick Lake, with a view into wooded hills and a western sky.

In early morning, I have watched the sun, like an artist, dipping his brush in scarlet paint, cover the hills with a warm and comforting wash of sunrise. As daylight reached the lake, I could see the twisted, whirling patterns of snow, as if a frenzied woman had tried to sweep it away. A great flock of evening grosbeaks emerged from the woods and hurried to the feeders happily greeting another day and a magnificent bald eagle sailed across the sky casting its shadow on the glittering ice. And another day was here!

It seemed no time until the sun had set, reaching its farthest point toward the western sky and turned the world into a kaleidoscope of rich golds, yellows and rose. Then night descended with its comforting arms of darkness. But, in the small hours of morning, sleepless, I returned to watch the night.

A thin sickle of moon was dipping down over the distant hills, and stars, bright and beautiful as a baby's eyes, twinkled in the dark, blue velvet of the heavens. And, gentle as a kiss, a shaft of brightness fell to earth, and almost as if in acknowledgment, I heard the mournful sound of a night bird.

Perhaps this was the time for a quiet prayer, but I have seldom been a silent prayer. As I looked out upon the majesty of that glorious sky, I could only hear the triumphant sounds of that great Mormon hymn, *All is Well ... All is Well.*

Flowers for Winter

I have been wondering why winter "blues" don't have too much effect upon me and I have come to the conclusion that it is because I love flowers and have many blossoming all winter in the house. At present there are daffodils, crocus, tulips, magnificent Amaryllis, one of which has two stems and seven very large blossoms, and various colors of hyacinths. I also have an hibiscus which produces a new scarlet blossom every day; and my pride and joy is a Bird of Paradise plant which produces at least two beautiful blossoms every winter. Where do I buy all these joy givers? I don't.

I often wonder why more people don't plant bulbs for winter blooming. Perhaps they think there is too much preparation, and this isn't so. Here are a few tips on planting flowers so you will have beauty from the first snow until Easter. Use two parts of good garden soil and one part peat moss and plant daffodils, narcissi, crocus, and tulips just below the surface of the soil. Put them in a cool, dark place for from three to five weeks. When you bring them into the house, keep as cool as possible for a while, then fertilize, water, and enjoy.

I grow hyacinths in glasses made for this purpose, fill the glass with water, put in cool, dark place for at least a month. When you bring them into the light of day, watch the blossoms emerge and smell the fragrance. I love Amaryllis, not only for their spectacular blossoms but for the sheer enjoyment of watching them grow, sometimes a half inch a day. These plants will bloom for you year after year.

When all danger of frost has gone, and the blooms have faded, the stalk should be cut off two inches above the bulb. Do not disturb the foliage. Place pot and all in the ground buried to top edge of the rim. Fertilize during the summer. In September bring into the house and do not water for about six weeks. Then fertilize, place in sunny window, and watch the miracle of a beautiful flowering plant.

❖

Using Our Senses

I know I regret my deteriorating sense of smell when trying to get the fragrance of my beautiful hyacinths, for I become more aware of my other senses—sight, hearing, taste, smell and touch. I wonder, however, if we really use those senses to their fullest extent?

I remember sitting on the porch one summer evening. I saw the night sky and a satellite that moved across the heavens at remarkable speed. I heard a coyote across the hills, and an owl with an almost similar call. I smelled the foliage of the trees as night dew laid its refreshing moisture on them. A night moth touched my hand and it was a pleasant sensation.

Do we really use our senses to the fullest? How often do our delicate taste buds take over? Roll the first strawberry from the garden across your tongue; spread homemade bread with good butter and savour the difference. Chew a sprig of watercress and enjoy the tartness. We sniff, but do we smell the earth after a summer shower, or appreciate the fragrance of lilacs in bloom.

Do we smell the earth as a farmer plows his field or slowly breathe in the headiness of home after a long absence. What do we really listen to? The racuous sounds of rock music or the soul-satisfying music of the great composers. Are we really familiar with the various cadences of bird song? What about the singing of insects on a warm, summer night, or the gentle lapping of water in a nearby stream.

Do we listen to those who call for help, the lonely, aged, the sick? How often have we touched the wings of a butterfly, or the feathers of a fallen bird, or caressed the skin of a newly bathed baby.

Happiness is found in the little things of life—things we too often overlook.

❖

Toad in the Hole

Have you ever seen a patrician nose wrinkle with distaste, and the owner of said proboscis back away as though he was smelling something foul? I had such a person around yesterday when I mentioned that I was making Toad in the Hole for dinner!

Of course, I could have invited him for dinner, given my pet Toad in the Hole a more elegant name, and his nose would have been spared that distorting wrinkle. Toad in the Hole is an old English dish made from thick slices of home-cured bacon, dipped in a good batter and deep fried, or just baked in a hot oven until cooked. Homemade applesauce or crab apple jelly is a good accompaniment.

I could have jolted the gentleman by offering him Pigs in a Blanket. Maybe he is more partial to pigs than toads. Perhaps I'd better give the readers the recipe. His Nibs will never know what he missed. This was a once-a-week dinner when I was a child and I still like it.

Cook until brown and almost done ten to twelve small links of sausage (that should serve four). Make a Yorkshire Pudding batter. Two well-beaten eggs; a pinch of salt; one cup of flour; and one cup of milk. Beat well. Pour into a well-greased dish or pan. Place sausages in batter. Bake in pre-heated oven at 450 degrees for fifteen minutes. Reduce heat to 350 and bake another fifteen minutes. The batter will rise, be beautifully brown, and taste excellent.

So! You wrinkle your nose! Go buy some hot dogs and put them on a soggy white bun.

❖

Beautiful Music

This afternoon, I spent a short time listening to beautiful music supplied by a group of birds in the pine trees. The words of poet Congreve came to mind. "Music hath charms to soothe a savage beast, to soften rocks, or bend a knotted oak." Surely Mr. Congreve was not referring to our present day rock music when he wrote those words.

When Billy Shakespeare wrote "The man that hath no music in himself, nor is not moved with concord of sweet sounds, is fit for treasons, stratagems and spoils," he had never tried sitting through a rock concert, nor was he watching a TV show expecting to listen to that kind of music which "heals a troubled soul." I can't imagine a world without music for it has always been a factor in my life from the time I was a child singing in the Sunday School Choir. I love good music and do have some good music piped into our living rooms from radio and television, however, the repetitive lyrics, insane gyrations and raucous sounds emanating from certain groups who seem to be so popular with the younger generation, remind me of the hospital wards where are housed slightly demented cases. The music is irritating, disoriented and just plain nauseous. That, by the way, is my opinion. There are, of course, people who go along and accept this type because it is "the thing to do." I am fortunate enough to have tapes made for me by my music-loving son-in-law, so I can enjoy Beethoven, Brahms, Chopin, and if I need music to ease my troubled mind, I choose Sibelius, Grieg and the beloved Dvorak.

Let me pay homage to the birds who begin life as the sun rises, and have the good sense to deliver comforting music with which to begin the day. "Such sweet, soft notes as yet musicians cunning never gave the enraptured air."

❖

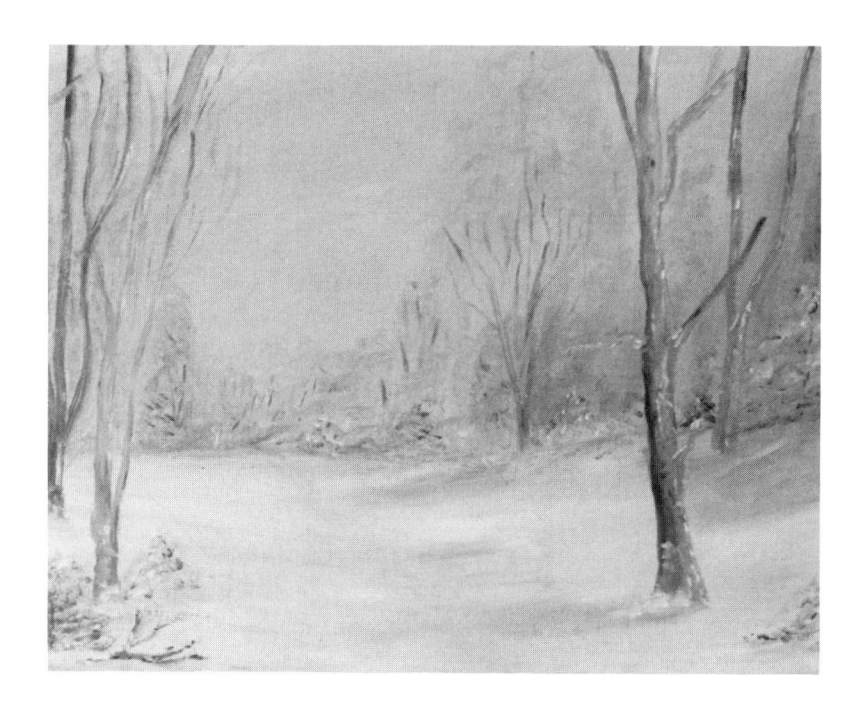

Winter Wonderland

The sun was rising above the snow-festooned pines and birds were assembling early around the feeders. I fixed a tray with fat and cereal, but before I could reach the feeder an eager chickadee alighted on my arm determined to be in the front line at breakfast.

There was peace, and a stillness that was heart-warming and comforting, and I almost purred with happiness.

The thermometer hovered around twenty degrees below zero as we started out on a short journey and snow crackled with staccato music beneath the car wheels. A deer crossed our path and rimed frost laced his nostrils, his eyes dilated with apprehension.

Each shrub beside the road had hanging necklaces of frost-coated cobwebs with designs no jeweler could copy. Smoke from chimneys made arches of mist across the road reminding me of fall fires and barbecues, and the fragrance of burning wood surpassed the pleasantness of fine, manmade perfume.

Dear Lord! What a world! The tops of tall trees reached heavenwards with their silver splendor, radiant against the cerulean blue of the morning sky—and my heart sang.

To live in such a world! Winter! Cold! tis true, but where else could life pick up such splendor with which to enrich our days?

❖

Your Work Is You

This is the time of year when we offer our congratulations to the young people who are graduating from high school. Many of these graduates are expecting to go on to college and perhaps wondering who will pay the tuition. If they are not wondering, then their parents certainly are, and with the economy as it is many parents will be unable to accept the obligation of high expenses. This leaves me wondering why the wish to rush off to college unless one is planning to enter the professional field.

Wouldn't a year of work, of learning to get along with people, no matter what their race, religion or economic status be a step towards higher education? It would certainly be enlightening what an eight hour day of work feels like and knowing there will be no excuse for neglecting to be on time or failure to show up for the job. It is true that we need professionals with a college background in such fields as medicine, electronics, science, etc., but who will fix our automobiles, repair the plumbing, paint the house or do carpentry? These artisans are important to our comfort and our health and their knowledge of the work in which they are engaged is profound. Let us not have too many people who consider themselves "over qualified" for the work they are doing. The most menial job has its value.

It was a wise man who said: "It is in making your work YOU. Put the stamp of your unique personality on the work you do. Pour your spirit into the talk. Make your work a reflection of your faith, your integrity, your ideals."

❖

Lavender

I just received a shipment of essential oils which I use in various hobbies. Because I love lavender I poured a few drops in a container atop the stove and the house is fragrant and takes my memories way back to the lovely village of Mitcham, in Surrey, England, where the finest lavender in the world is grown.

Lavender is a fragrance high in memory-content for most of us. Remember the lavender scented sheets on grandmother's four poster bed that sheltered us on our childhood visits? Balm to our bodies and wings to our dreams! Then, the fragrance of lavender meant security and simplicity as well as freshness and cleanliness. In fact, the botanical name, lavendula was derived from the Latin word, lavare, meaning "to wash." One of my first recollections of this clean fragrance, was the smell of the ladies as they walked into church on sunday mornings. One knew what they kept in their glove and handkerchief boxes!

But the use of lavender goes back much farther than grandmother's time. The ancient Romans used lavender lavishly in their famous baths, but probably in a dried form, for it wasn't until the 12th century that lavender water was invented. It is thought to have originated with Saint Hildegard of Bingen, a German Benedictine nun who was born in 1898 and whose cloister was in the Rhine valley. She was especially respected for her skill with medicines, so it is to be presumed she used lavender water in her medicines. In Spain it was used to heal wounds.

The lavender oil itself is obtained by distillation. The reaping of the flowers is, like that of many other flowers, a family industry in France. After harvesting, the flowers must be transported quickly to the distilleries which are near a village or a brook or well, where there is water for distillation. So, if you would like to take a trip down memory lane—try lavender!

❖

Early American Herb Recipes

Yesterday I found occasion to read a book which was given to me some time ago. The title is *Early American Herb Recipes* and the first item to amuse me was a Quaker doctor's description of prevailing practice: "When patients come to me, I, physics, bleeds, and sweat 'em; then, if they choose to die, what's that to I—I let's 'em."

Naturally, I wished to read some of the recipes. *Piles*: tea made of slippery elm is good for piles, and for humors of the blood; to be drank plentifully; Year 1838. *Nosebleed*: The bruised flowers of Ladies Bedstraw pushed up the nostrils stayeth their bleeding; Year 1652. *Wrinkles*: the juice of cowslip flowers is suggested for wrinkles. We say that they will and therefore cause the skin to smooth; Year 1629. *Headache*: the flowers of chamomile boiled in lee, are good to wash the head and comfort both it and the brain; Year 1652. *Asthma*: taken in meat, Saffron causes a long and easy breathing and helpeth the asthma: Year 1577. *Dropsy*: Parsley is good for dropsy, gravel, and obstruction of the liver and kidneys; Year 1814. *Salad*: Nasturtiums are now become an acceptable Sallat, as well the leaf as the blossom; Year 1677.

If you have received a rabbit from a hunter and would like an old fashioned recipe for cooking, here is a 1668 recipe.

Roast Rabbit: When you have cased the rabbits, skewer their heads with their mouths upon their backs, stick their forelegs into their ribs. Skewer the hind legs doubled, then make a pudding for them with the crumbs of half a loaf of bread, a little parsley, margoram and thyme. Mix them into a light stuffing with half pound of butter and two eggs and bake.

Want to try it? How many forelegs does a rabbit have?

❖

Laughter

What is there about laughter that affects the entire body? Tenseness disappears, sadness slips into the distance and even pain seems to subside. Laughter is just a bubble that rises from the throat and yet it can perform miracles. How many times have you known a short chuckle of laughter put an end to an uncomfortable argument? Inject laughter into tense situations to save the day; laughter calms tempers and soothes jangled nerves.

I can take my memory back 70 years and see my first exhibit of the power of laughter. There was an elderly woman in our small village who had endured more tragic experiences than she could take, so she decided to end it all. It was when she was fashioning a loop in a rope with which to hang herself that a young man appeared at the door of the barn. "That, my friend, is too big a loop for your skinny neck" he said laughingly. The old lady looked at him and began to laugh. The rope was thrown away; the boy put his arm around her shoulder and they walked away laughing. I remember wondering if the flowers along the garden path were also laughing.

Have you ever watched the weary look on the face of some elderly people as they push their grocery cart around the super market? They arrive at the checkout counter, and the cashier, with a beautiful smile, says "good morning." Weary faces light up as though a ray of sunshine had just caught them. I am often asked, "What will remove wrinkles from the face of the elderly"? "Why try to remove them; they are laughter lines" is my usual response.

Hufeland made this remark. "Laughter is a most healthful exertion; it is one of the greatest helps to digestion with which I am acquainted; and the custom prevalent among our forefathers, of exciting it at table by jesters and buffoons, was founded on true medical principles."

❖

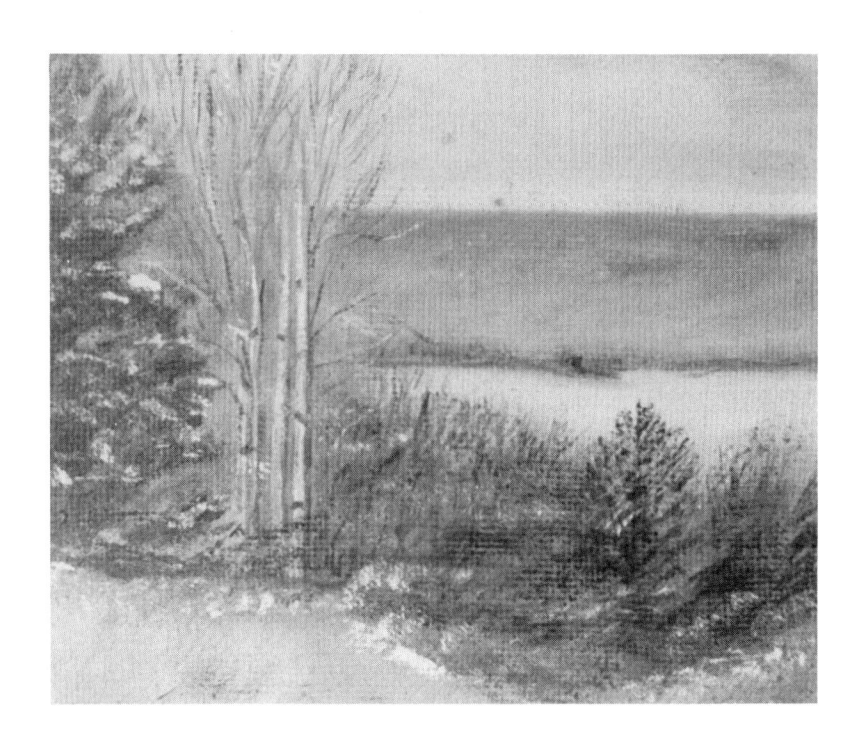

Fairyland

I don't believe I'd enjoy missing Winter in our north country for I like the everyday change in the weather. Waking up to face a world changed to fairyland with every tree and twig laced with an elegant hoar frost, and the rising sun making magic of the distant hills. Patterns of frost on the window pane with designs no artist seems able to copy. Where else can one observe the antics of squirrels around a bird feeder fending off with authority the waiting birds, or watch a large flock of evening grosbeaks claiming first chance at the suet and sunflower dining shelf.

It was a delightful experience to observe yesterday, five partridge pecking a few crab apples left on a tree below our window, while, on the ground, an amorous male bird spread his wings and muttered sweet nothings to the "hard to catch," indifferent females.

There are flocks of small birds either optimistic about Spring or are on their way to summer quarters. They are most polite, just gathering from the ground the sweet morsels dropped by greedy blue jays, then they fly to nearby branches and sing their paean of thanks.

Today the wind has made geometric patterns across the lake and graceful otters are playing tag at the mouth of the stream, while a large collection of newly arrived crows announce their presence with raucous calls. The snow made a musical, crunchy sound as I walked my mile and a half today and I began to sing an almost forgotten Irish melody that satisfied my mood. If the deer objected, they kept a safe distance and the world around me, with its pristine beauty was very satisfying.

There's a wind making its own special music, and I swear I heard a robin. Soon Spring will awaken the earth and once again life begins anew with the pulsing sounds that herald the bursting of buds and the beginning of life for the dormant hills.

❖

No One Listens to Me

I remember my Irish Granny giving advice to a sick man, "God cures sick people, doctors take the credit. Don't fasten your thoughts on yourself, try pleasing others." A while ago, as I stood looking at a group of young people, I wondered where they would be five years from now—on their way to achieving their ambitions or relying on drugs to give them support? Adults are not the only ones to have tension headaches, stomach aches, and an increase in blood pressure. A hurried child may also show these symptoms. Some of these upsets are based on parental separation, divorce and a pressing need to excel academically. In the rush of everyday affairs, parents are sometimes too concerned with their own problems, or to keep the family afloat financially to stop and realize the same insecurity and fears they are battling are affecting their children. Most parents try to do a good job and are well intentioned and love their children, but when under stress it is difficult for them to decenter themselves, and so they also stress their children.

In today's economic state, many families find it necessary for both parents to be wage-earners. What happens when a child goes home to an empty house? Will they be content knowing that when Mother and Dad come home they can all share the day's happenings? Will there be loving hugs and words of encouragement? Will Mother and Dad take the time to listen to their son or daughter as they recount their concerns, or are the parents afraid to express their love with a kiss, a hug and a word of praise?

Why do I concern myself with these problems? Because when I work with the committee for drug abuse the most common complaint of the drug abusing children was "No one ever listens to me."

Don't be afraid to hug and to listen; children have feelings, too.

Beautiful Skin

It is about this time of year when we look in the mirror and wonder what happened to our moist skin and observe with concern the extra wrinkles that hot, dry heating has brought us. I was given a beautiful very comprehensive herb book at Christmastime and I found some great recipes which may prevent us from turning the mirror to the wall.

The author does, however, warn that "the health and appearance of the skin reflects the inner physical and psychological health of an individual." Healthy skin and hair cannot be obtained by cosmetic use alone and attention should be paid to well-balanced diet and adequate exercise, rest and general health. Herbal or natural cosmetics are, however, of material benefit to the body especially if used on a regular basis. Since the author, Malcolm Stewart, is considered one of the finest herbologists in the country, I don't hesitate to pass along some of his ideas.

Eye Bath: A quick and simple remedy for eye strain requires placing a slice of cucumber over each eye and resting in a darkened room for five to ten minutes. Be sure your cucumber is fresh and never use the same slice twice. *Black heads*: Blackheads are a problem even on an otherwise unblemished skin. Rub the blemished spot with a slice of tomato! *Face Mask*: Beat an egg white, add the juice of a lemon, or vinegar or buttermilk. Spread over entire face and allow to dry. Rinse off with tepid water and apply cold cream. Another mask recipe is: Two whipped egg whites, one cucumber and a teaspoonful of lemon juice. Put everything in the electric blender and spread over face until dry. OR—for dry skin, oatmeal makes a fine base and bleaches the skin. Mix with your favorite flower water, such as rose water or elder flower water. For old gals—like me, there is an anti-wrinkle cream. Drop ten poppy blossom petals in 10 ounces of boiling water and allow it to stand one hour. Apply to face. Hail to beauty!

❖

A Smile, a Laugh

How many people know the value of a smile? It is one of our most valuable assets. It can change a plain face into one of beauty; push a look of sadness into oblivion; turn tears into laughter and sadness into happiness. Even a scolding doesn't leave resentment, if there's a smile on the face of the scolder. Have you ever walked up to a check-out counter in a store with a complaint on your lips, only to be met with a smiling clerk who says, "Good morning." Whatever happened to your complaint? A smile pushes wrinkles into the category of laughter lines, and brings a frightened child into the shelter of your arms.

I well remember a customer who came into my drug store many times a week. Her expression was sad, sullen and woebegone and none enjoyed waiting on her. One day I decided to leave the prescription room and greet her with a smile. It took a bit of conversation and a lot of smiling. And then it worked! It was almost miraculous to discover that underneath dourness there was beauty, light, even an expression of happiness. I remembered the words of Henry Ward Beecher, "A man without mirth is like a wagon without springs. . . he is jolted disagreeably by every pebble in the road."

A smile! It will lighten your own life as well as others. Don't you feel like buying more goods when the clerk who is waiting on you wears a smile? That "have a good day" comment by a clerk without a smile is as uninteresting as a "kiss without a moustache" to use one on my Granny's expressions. Laughter calms tempers and soothes jangled nerves. Laughter is the best medicine for a long and happy life. He who laughs . . . lasts.

❖

Freezing Herbs

"How can I preserve herbs so I can use them during the winter?" This is a question I am often asked, so perhaps I can tell you how I manage to have herbs to flavor food instead of salt which is taboo in our diet.

Many cooks prefer freezing fresh herbs because the process is quick and the herbs, when thawed, have a close-to-fresh flavor. Cut the herbs in the morning when the oils have built up and the flavor is at its best. If you have some plants that are late and not fully matured, just cut the leaves that are a few inches high and use them. I find that they give the best flavor.

Wash the herbs thoroughly to remove dust and splashings of dirt but do use cold water, for hot water will destroy those aromatic oils which are essential for flavor.

Lightly press the herbs between paper towels until almost free of moisture. Remove any woody stems or discolored leaves.

I then make bouquets garnis and put them in small plastic bags (these are to drop into soups and stews to give flavor and are than removed) or I chop them and pack in plastic containers. Or—chop and put into ice trays, freeze them and transfer to containers. A little water must be added to the herbs in ice trays. If you are going to use a liquid such as chicken stock then just pack the herbs in chicken stock and ice-tray freeze. Half the soup job is done!

Always thaw herbs at room temperature and *never refreeze*.

We used to feel that it wasn't possible to cook—with taste—unless the salt box was near at hand, but today, with blood pressure victims advised to eliminate salt from their diet, a much better way has been found to give flavor to the most gourmet type of food. And once herbs are used in place of salt, the smart cook will put the salt out in the garden to put on the tails of the snails. Happy cooking!

❖

Children

A few days ago I sat drinking coffee with a friend who is also a grandmother and, as is usual with grandmothers, the subject was grandchildren.

My friend had raised four children on a farm, children who had gone on to college and become wonderful, useful citizens. I have never believed fully in the idea that the character of a person depended entirely upon heredity and environment. Love, parental understanding, pride in achievement, these are some of the essentials for character building.

As I listened to my companion, I wondered how many children were denied the privilege of touching an animal, listening to the sounds of nature, smelling the odor of a barn and inhaling the fragrance of foliage. How many had witnessed the birth of a calf or a lamb, or observed the building of a bird's nest.

Perhaps these experiences are some of the things our young people are missing, and, being deprived of the things nature has to offer, they turn to other forms of excitement—not guaranteed to build character.

"My children would beg to have a picnic in the barn on a rainy day because they loved the sound of rain on the tin roof. Their drink was rain water caught in a cup from the dripping eaves because it was the "best ever." Then she continued "We weeded the fields together and walked the hedgerows in a fall, gathering berries for pies, jams and jellies." Somehow, after she left, I found myself being projected into the lives of these children, realizing that the tasks given on the farm, were privileges denied my child. These wonderful joys of achievement were the character builders that resulted in good citizenship. Perhaps as parents we have overlooked the simple things of life and have been too generous in bestowing the luxuries of affluence which have little value as character-builders.

❖

Juneberries

The ripe fruits of the Juneberries hang like purple jewels from the trees, almost begging to be gathered. Although they have ten large seeds, they add flavor to the fruit and when they are cooked, they become soft and lend a lovely almond taste to the cooking. I enjoy the fruit straight from the tree, but when cooked and a little acid added such as vinegar or lemon juice, they are delicious.

Dried they can be used all winter as currants or raisins in fruit cake, rice pudding, etc. If you would rather can them, here is a recipe: Bring to a boil two cups of water and four cups of sugar (or two of honey). Carefully pour in six cups of Juneberries and simmer for two minutes. Stir in three tablespoons of lemon juice. Pack in hot sterile jars. Cover with hot, juicy syrup. Seal and process for twenty minutes in water bath.

Canned berries make superior pies, although one can also use fresh fruit. Mix four cups ripe berries with one and one-fourth cups sugar or half as much honey. Add four tablespoons melted butter and two tablespoons of lemon juice. Pour into crust, top with another crust and bake in moderate oven for about fifty minutes.

If you like jam you will enjoy Juneberry jam. Put the washed fruit through a medium fine food chopper. Then measure four cups and add just enough water to cover, and simmer until the berries are tender and pulpy. Add three cups sugar and the juice of two lemons, the shredded pulp of two oranges with all the pulp and the grated rind. Let it bubble gently until it sets— about half an hour, do use these berries when making muffins.

Try one of my favorites. Put berries, as many as you wish, in the bottom of a flat casserole dish and sweeten with whatever you like. Add lemon juice and pour over a popover batter and bake. Anyway—try some of these fruits of the field and forget some of the junk items we are urged to eat.

❖

Vinegar, The Workhorse

Vinegar! It is the workhorse of the kitchen. It stops the advance of a cold sore, kills the sting of an insect bite and removes the calcium deposits in my pots and pans. It is needed for pickling, preserving, tenderizing tough meat and chicken and adds a sour pungency to dishes ranging from vinegar pie to tomato ketchup. None can say when vinegar first came into use. It was old when Ruth, in the Bible, dipped her morsel of bread into the vinegar and Caesar's legions mixed it with drinking water. It was probably discovered by ancient peoples accidentally along with wine.

Yeast and bacteria are ever present in the air, too small to be seen by the naked eye. Perhaps some of these yeasts fell by accident into uncovered earthenware jars and caused the juice to ferment and become wine, and in time the bacteria dropped into the wine and soured it and so became vinegar. Although it started with wine, imaginative cooks throughout the world have invented many variants such as banana vinegarrice and honey vinegar and even brandy.

The English, years ago, began to apply malt in an effort to dispose of stale ale and beer and today, they still like malt vinegar best.

Many famous chefs employ vinegar with herbs for making remarkable sauces and for marinating meats. The strangest of all uses was employed by a gang of thieves looting Marseilles during the Black Plague in the Middle Ages. They choked down a mixture of cloves, sage, rosemary, rue and vinegar in the belief that this hair-raising brew would protect them from disease. But even they seem unimaginative when compared to Cleopatra who made vinegar history on the night when she dissolved a perfect pearl in vinegar and drank it down with a flourish to show Mark Anthony that she could consume a fortune in one meal.

I will still use white vinegar as the workhorse and keep the cider vinegar for sauces.

❖

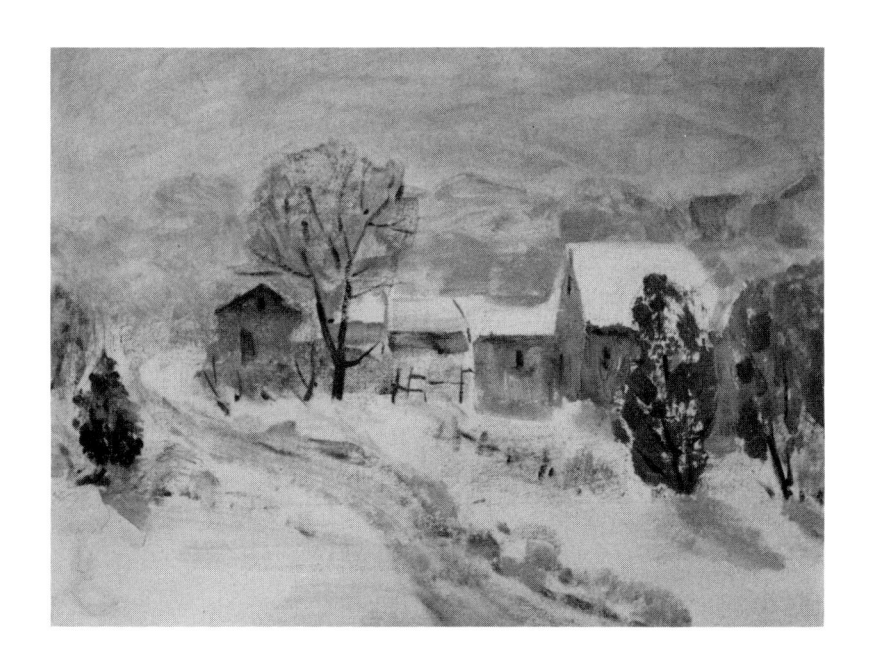

Beauty in Winter

No one likes the ice or the deep snow, but who doesn't enjoy the beauty only winter in our North Country can give us. It was zero on this particular morning and I watched the sunrise turn the hills to a warm maroon. There was a hoar frost and every twig was covered with a pristine whiteness. The nine foot wire fence around the vegetable garden was indescribable with design, and the night winds had whipped the snow into geometrical patterns across the lawn.

I recognized the tracks of the animals who had foraged for food in the shadow of night. Deer, a stray cat, squirrels rising early for food donations. The huge tracks of a jack rabbit and the mixed marks left by many birds. And, of course, the feeders were empty. As I looked through the duskiness of the woods, there were prisms of dancing lights like twinkling stars. I knew I wasn't in heaven, for who smells bacon and eggs in heaven? But those flashing lights intrigued me, so I watched.

I saw birds fly to a bush, and, as they landed or flew away, the icy fragments moved, caught the light and flashed those mysterious prisms into the winter wonderland. The greenhouse windows were covered with a frosty magic of patterns with no repetition of design, and, as I watched the dawn light disappear, a pale sun turned the world to wonderland. The frosty whiteness was now a pale pink, like the frosting on a child's birthday cake. Dark blue shadows spread out from the trees along the shore line and chickadees called out to tell me the time was *now!* I scattered sunflower seeds and was thanked most vocally. In less than five minutes they were all there—chickadees, evening grosbeaks, blue jays and squirrels on the outer edge of the breakfast spread. And, as I watched, observing no malice, enmity, or jealousy, I wished we humans could copy some of the characteristics of these small creatures.

❖

Mistletoe

Can you remember the first time you were kissed under the mistletoe? I can; and I was sure the kisser would ask me to marry him, but he married somone else. He really had no taste.

Mistletoe, so much in evidence at Christmastime, is a parasite and belongs to the Loranthaceae family, of which there are almost 1,500 species, most of which are parasitic. Mistletoe may vary according to the host plant on which it is found, although it seems to prefer the apple tree. The ancient Druids believed that the drug obtained from this plant was more potent if the mistletoe grew on an oak.

Mistletoe is presently being examined for possible anti-cancer effects. It contains substances called lecithins which may combine with certain cancer cells; the chemistry and pharmacology of the plant is very complicated however, and no definite results have yet been demonstrated in humans. It is however, used in combination with other drugs to treat hypertension, and associated nervous complaints.

There are many legends about this ancient herb. Most churches in old England wouldn't allow it inside their doors because of its pagan connections. But priests of the ancient world, the Druids, once held the mistletoe so sacred that it could only be gathered by the head Arch Druid who cut it from its nest in the oak tree with a silver sickle.

It was also believed by the early Christians that the wood from a mistletoe tree formed the cross on which Christ was crucified and that, as punishment the plant was forever doomed to be a parasite.

The Scandinavians, who left behind much of their folklore and traditions, had their own view of the merits of this plant. According to custom, if two enemies met casually or accidentally under a plant of mistletoe in the forest, they were required to lay down their weapons and call a truce until the next day. Culpeper's Complete Herbal states that mistletoe is under the dominion of the sun. Well—it's kissing time!

My Dream Harvest

They are all here—eleven of them. Seed catalogues! With mountains of snow piled up around me and not an inch of garden in sight, I sit and drool!

Huge, red tomatoes with never a blemish, beans, to be gathered by the bushel in just a few minutes. Cucumbers too polite to create even a gentle burp; potatoes that make me dream of new peas and tiny spuds in an elegant sauce. They are all here in brilliant colors and emphatic statements regarding their authenticity.

I persuade my husband to write down the items as I check them off. Beets, pea pods, lettuce—on and on. Of course there are interruptions such as; "Why three kinds of lettuce?" Or "What's the difference in carrots. Wouldn't just one kind be enough?" "Remember what happened to that new kind of beet you tried last year?"

I quietly ignore all remarks and proceed with my checking.

It was when I was in the marigold department, and I'll admit I was slightly carried away, and who wouldn't be with all those colors from which to choose. Imagine those glorious yellows and reds and golds with maybe a few creamy ones interspersed here and there. But was there reason for my husband's remark as he put his pen away.

"Good heavens! Are you off your rocker! You're up to fifty dollars right now. Better sleep on it. Maybe tomorrow you'll be more sane."

Ha! Just wait til I harvest all those beautiful vegetables!!

❖

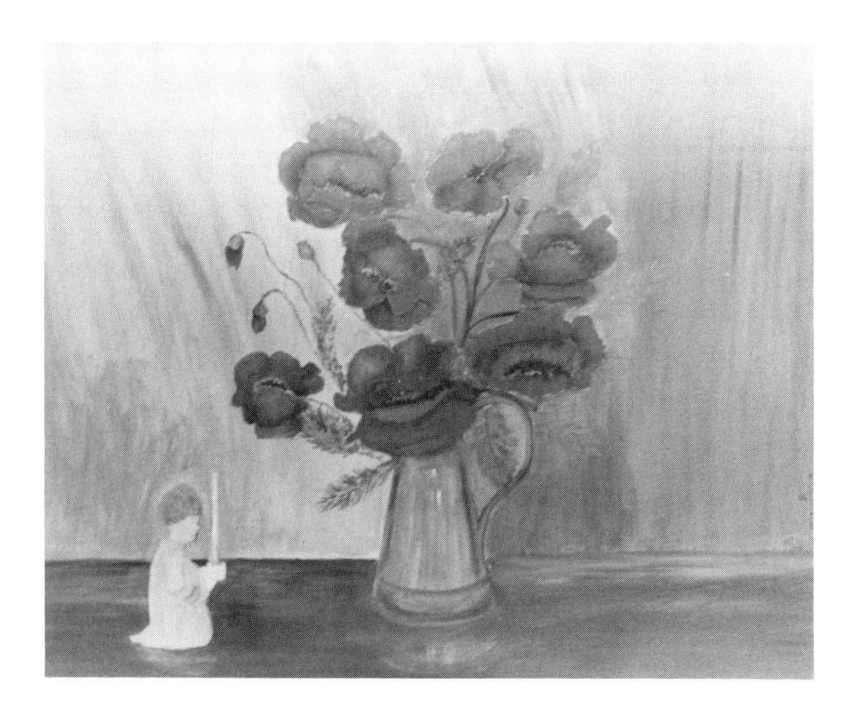

Christmas

What is Christmas? It is the day we celebrate the birth of Jesus. A day of happiness and rejoicing. Christmas is celebrated in many different ways in many countries and, almost always, there is the Christmas tree.

Many scholars believe the Christmas tree began in ancient Rome. It appears in Germany in 1604, so ancient literature informs us. Tree worship was common in Scandinavian countries and to this day the Swedes and Norwegians place a small fir tree on the ridge pole of a newly-built home for good luck.

One legend tells us how the first Christmas tree was miraculously revealed on Christmas Eve, twelve hundred years ago.

Winfred, an Englishman who had gone to Germany to spread the teachings of Jesus, found a group of worshipers gathered at the Oak of Geismar about to sacrifice little Prince Asult to the god of Thor. Winfred stopped the sacrifice, and cut down the "blood oak." As it fell, a young fir tree appeared. The missionary then told the people that the fir tree was the Tree of Life or of Christ.

The years have passed. The days when we hung up a stocking on Christmas Eve and were delighted when we found an orange, a pencil, or if we were lucky, a hair ribbon, on Christmas morning are long gone. Today, harassed men and women search the stores for gifts they can ill afford in order to appease the wishes of family and friends. Somehow, along the way, we have forgotten the gift of love—a gift that can be made every day of the year. The word, the letter, the smile, the unexpected gift which comes with frequency to lighten and brighten the heart of the lonely. What is Christmas? It is 365 days each year remembering the teachings of Christ and being a good human being. Did not Jesus say, "Do unto others as you would have them do unto you..."

"Dear Santa:

Put into my stocking a dash of human kindness. Add some of the breath of vision that will make me realize that, in truth, I am my brother's keeper. Pour in some oil of graciousness—the mark of a true human. Give me the opportunity to play my part in this big, busy world, and to regulate my life that, when I pass on, no man can say of me, 'he lived for self alone.'

Leave me a generous package of good cheer, so that when my neighbor is weighed down with despair, I may go to help him look up and have hope anew. Bring me a jack-in-the-box like the one that thrilled my childish heart.

Make all the children glad but do not forget the grownups who have relinquished the carefreeness of youth for the stern realities of the daily struggles. Write upon their minds and hearts the message that real happiness consists in service to one's fellows, not in things for oneself."

Happy Christmas! May God hold you in the palm of his hand.

❖

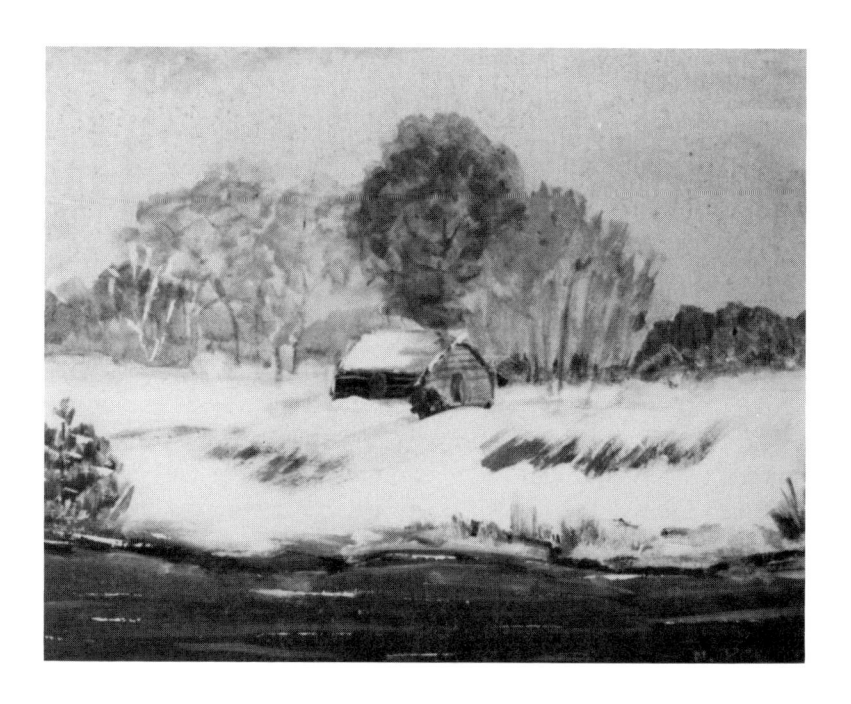

The Wood Stove

There's a fire burning in the wood stove in my kitchen. How often I have been tempted to discard that space-occupying piece of cast iron, and how happy I am to have its warmth on such a day as this.

The fragrance of wood smoke, of bread freshly baked in its huge oven, parsley drying on wire racks with thyme and sweet marjoram to keep company. With the door slightly open, the pungent fragrance fills every corner of the house. No need for artificial deodorizers to remove house odors!

I have lines strung in most unusual places and they are filled with small bunches of herbs drying and readying for winter use. There's the sharpness of sweet basil which will be married to every tomato dish and which will enhance the variety of omelettes made for breakfast this winter.

Mints, delicate and beautiful: orange, pineapple and apple, all of which delight the palate of the gourmet. They also make excellent jellies, turn a fruit salad into ambrosia, and chopped, add distinction to tossed salads of any kind.

Something different, and good, is apple-mint butter. One tablespoon of chopped parsley and two tablespoons of chopped apple mint worked into a half pound of good butter. Use on crackers, hot biscuits, or over cooked green beans or cauliflower.

I have gathered oregano, leaving enough for the bees who buzz around it in swarms. The oregano I grow is generally known as wild marjoram, and while it can be used medicinally, it enhances the flavor of many foods. It is indispensible to the Latin and Oriental cooks. Put it in marinades for all meats, in stuffings for such elegant fare as cabbage leaves in which are rolled ground meat and rice simmered in consomme. And the most beautiful winter bouquets can be made from the dark purple-red blossoms which are now at their best. Today summer savory was cut and brought in to dry, and there's an almost intoxicating perfume in the house. The beautiful herbs!

Experiment, but be careful, for too much herb, as too much of anything, can be discouraging.

❖

Kindness

We are a complaining, critical people. Perhaps that is good, for it comes with that freedom for which we should all be grateful. The freedom to express our feelings openly without fear of reprisal. We have had much to criticize, tis true, but we have also had much for which to be thankful and grateful. And now we have a new year. A time to review the things that have happened—and to bitch about the future, if that is the mood. It is also time to turn over the coin and look for some of the good things—the wonderful benefits afforded us in this land of the free. And wouldn't we all feel better if we did just that?

I well remember some words being written by a poet with whom I was working at a writers conference one time. "Let me be a little kinder, let me be a little blinder to the faults of those around us." In 1979 we might be happier if we followed that advice. Another poet, Ella Wheeler Wilcox, gave us a poem to live with in the coming year:

> As the old year sinks down in time's ocean
> Stand ready to launch with the new
> And waste no regrets, no emotion,
> As the spars and the masts pass from view.
> Weep not if some treasures go under,
> And sink in the other ship's hold—
> That new year that's sailing just yonder
> May bring you more good than the old.
> Throw overboard useless regretting,
> Or deeds which you cannot undo,
> And learn the great art of forgetting
> Old things which embitter the new.
> Sing who will of dead years departed,
> I shun them and bid them adieu,
> And the song that I sing happy hearted,
> Is a song of the glorious new!

Happy New Year!

A Zest for Life

Sitting quietly in the evening twilight, I was abruptly asked what it was like to have lived for 84 years and what changes have taken place in the world during those years.

I should begin by saying I'm a happy, healthy woman with a zest for life and an interest in people. Having lived through more than three-quarters of this century, I have been privileged to experience progress so remarkable it was science fiction just a short time ago.

I've savored most all of the emotions known to a human... hunger, aloneness, pain, sorrow, joy, love and lasting friendships. I nursed the wounded in World War I, and, as a pharmacist, I have learned the art of listening and of empathy.

Sure I have weaknesses—lots of 'em. A black cat scares the bejabbers out of me, and I do believe in ghosts. If you have ever spent a night in one of the old ancestral houses in England or Ireland you would too! Superstitious? Yes! I have a silver dime dated 1910 and I have used it to wish on the new moon for many years. That's why I get a crick in my neck at times—just looking for the blessed thing. When I turn over that dime I make a wish, not for myself, or it would never come true.

I have learned to distinguish between the wheat and the chaff. I know that love and friendship cannot be bought but must be earned every day.

There are so many things I still want to do, I have decided to live a few more years. I want to sit beside my love in the cool of the evening . . . to watch the sunset and the rise of the moon and to ask what my husband would like for breakfast—and try to change his mind.

These words come to my mind:

> Steady my hurried pace with the vision of the eternal reach of time. Give me, amid the confusion of the day, the calmness of the everlasting

hill. Teach me the art of taking minute vacations—of slowing down to look at a flower, to chat with a friend, to pat a dog, to read a few lines from a good book. Slow me down, Lord, and inspire me to send my roots deep into the soil of life's enduring values that I may grow toward the stars of my greater destiny.

——— ❖ ———

❖

The Boy with the Pipe

A Christmas story by Nellie Poulsen, from her early days as a pharmacist

I think of him as the boy with the pipe. A boy with a dog is a pretty common thing, but whoever associates a boy with a pipe. I used to see him standing there after school let out, just looking. He never disturbed anyone, never riffled the funny books as so many children do, or talked, or leaned too closely against the candy case lending suspicion. No, he just stood there, a little on tip-toe and looked.

I judged him to be about eight years old. He was mighty lean where a boy of eight ought to be filling out, and he had the brown, straight, unruly hair that is the despair of doting mothers. Across his little turned up nose there was a sprinkle of freckles that gave him a look of pertness and in a way attracted him to me. One day I got curious and walked over to him.

"Oh, it's a pipe, eh, sonny?" I queried.

"Yes, that one. Could I please see it?"

I opened the case to take out the pipe he indicated and put it into his boyish hands. perhaps I smiled as I saw the gestures he used in looking it over. He examined it carefully for flaws in the wood, sniffed at it, took it apart to see how it worked and last of all—you guessed it—he stuck it between his teeth, or rather where his teeth should have been, because he was at the between-teeth age.

"Good piece of briar," I ventured haphazardly and he rewarded me with a pitying look, the result, I found out afterwards, of my inability to distinguish between briar and . . .

Next day he wasn't back, or the next. Then I looked up one afternoon to see him standing in his usual place at the back of the door, hands thrust deep into his trouser pockets, his eyes glued to that pipe. I noticed that in between earnest gazes at the beloved pipe, I was the recipient of a few of those looks. I smiled and went about my work. Usually it is the older editions who pass their smiles across the counter, and then, only until they have felt the keen edge of my tongue. But here he was, standing all at once at my prescription counter, eyes as big as saucers, his cheeks a little pink from excitement.

"That pipe, Miss. Do you suppose I could buy it if I paid a dime a week?"

A dime a week. Well, that's what I call deferred payment all right. But right then I would gladly have given him the pipe.

"Certainly," was all I said.

"You see, it is ten weeks until Christmas and I can have it paid for by that time," he had it all figured out, so I took the pipe from the case, put it in the box that was built for the five dollar pipe, and wrapped it up.

"Your name, please."

"Jon Thomas, and please don't put an H in the John."

Little old man spelling his name to me, a thin dime held preciously between his thumb and forefinger, I wondered who he might be and wanted to know. But I don't ask these little boys questions about themselves. One just treats them as you might their elders, respectfully, equally. Anyway that's what I did.

"It won't be sold now, will it?" he asked eagerly.

"Not for all the tea in China," I answered and left him standing there.

He didn't come back until the next payment was due. Then I met him half way down the store for I knew he had the dime and wanted to be treated as a real customer. If his mouth watered at the sight of the candy bars he brushed elbows with, he never gave any sign. He just watched me gravely, as I gave him credit on the back of his package, and was off across the vacant lot.

Payments were made regularly each week and it needed two weeks until Christmas. Things began to hum in the corner drug store and somehow I lost count of time. Then when I was passing the pipe case one day, I happened to think of the boy. It was with a feeling of shock that I noticed no payment had been made for two weeks and I wondered what catastrophy had occurred to keep that boy from buying his pipe.

I stood talking to one of my local customers at the door the next day. That was when I heard all about Jon. We saw him passing on the other side of the street.

"Do you know that boy?" I asked her.

"Oh, yes, that is Jon Thomas." She laughed remembering. "Funny thing. He came and begged me to let him keep my sidewalks clean of snow all winter for a dime a week."

"Yes?" and there was urgency in my word.

"Well, we had a lot of snow for a few weeks, you remember, and for the last two weeks there hasn't been any. Poor Jon, he is always looking at the sky to see whether snow is coming." She laughed at that, but, you see, she didn't have any children.

I heard the rest of the story from someone else. Jon's father was a paralytic, getting well, but very slowly. Jon adored him, even more so than the mother who went out daily to work in order to keep her little family going.

Snow began to fall that night and it had been years since we had had such a storm. Next morning was Saturday and no school for Jon. I sent the fountain boy to tell him that I'd like to see him about a little job. He came, not because he expected work. It was the thought of the pipe, I knew, that gave him that look of fearfulness. His words tumbled out before I had even reached the place where he stood.

"It is snowing, Miss, and I'll be able to pay for it. Don't sell it, please."

I got over the lump in my sentimental woman's throat, and managed to say, "I want you to clean my sidewalks for me, Jon, if you will. There's quite a lot and it's a big job, Jon." I wished he wouldn't look at me like that, eyes bright and his mouth open even so slightly to better hear to whatever else I had to say.

"It is worth fifty cents, I'd say," I went on, "You could clean the windows afterwards and make it an even dollar."

He didn't say anything, just stood.

"Well, what about it? Want the job?" I asked a little sharply.

He was off across the lot, his heels almost touching his head as he sped homeward to get the snow shovel.

No, he wasn't overpaid. That was some job for an eight year old. I watched him, saw his thin shoulder blades push out under the weight of the snow and his breath labor in his little chest. He rested for a minute between snow and windows but was on the job and doing it well the next time I looked.

He didn't take the dollar. Instead he bought his mother a dollar bottle of cologne which had somehow been reduced in price and paid the balance on the pipe. I wrapped it in Christmas paper and tied it with ribbon, red on the package for his dad and blue for his mother. He took them in his hands, blistered from the shovel and held them as though they were the most precious things on earth.

Have you ever seen a little boy with red in his cheeks, run his tongue across his lips because they were burning up with an inner joy? I have.

——— ❖ ———

So, You'd Like to Fill a Prescription!

DON'T . . . if you have the facility for tossing together a good batch of pancakes or stirring up a pound of homemade cold cream, get it into your head that the Lord intended you to take up pharmacy for a living. There's more to it than stirring and rolling. Mixing might be a better word since you are the things being mixed and your own ability to come out right side up depends upon your mastery to be able to take it.

Being Irish with a dash of Scotch, and a woman to boot, I am almost immune to the assumptions of my fellowman when he imagines that being a pharmacist is merely a matter of oil and attar of roses. That is, I should be immune, after twenty-five years of trying to convince the public—the man end of it anyway—that a woman might accidentally have a few brains, for the exertion has somewhat deadened the feeling part of me.

Then, when I hear these poor dear workers groaning about their forty hour week, I do a little quick mental arithmetic. That's the one time when I pull in my midriff and inflate my chest for I know they couldn't endure my seventy-five hours,—and live.

Some sweet young thing, all golden hair and blue eyes, opened the door yesterday and dilating her sensitive nostrils, murmured,

"I just love the smell of a drug store. Someday I am going to be a pharmacist. It's such pleasant work."

I unkinked my back, got the ashes out of my voice, and decided then and there that I would keep a record of one day in a drug store for the benefit of just such innocent young things. It went something like this, —

Seven thirty. My guess is that the man who made alarm clocks famous was never a victim of his own invention. Oh, well, fifteen minutes in which to dress and ten for my orange juice. Luxurious leisure! If only I don't hug the bed until it is too late for anything to eat.

Eight o'clock. I insert the key in the drug store door.

"Stamps!" It sounds like a general issuing a command, but it is two hundred pounds of indignation because the stamp machine has been moved a foot and the lady cannot see it.

Tobacco, matches, papers, change for the telephone! A red lolypop for a curly haired cherub. It must be red!

"Operator, operator! You didn't return my dime." Then ensues an argument until I had a chance to show the angry customer the return box with her shining dime lying at the bottom.

"Will you do something for my child's arm?" asks a worried mother with her eight year old. I took a look at the pus sack hanging from the wrist and another from the elbow and suggested a doctor at once. She argued that she had no money for doctors and that was her reason for coming to me, and anyhow, she said that the child had had it for a week, so she guessed it might be all right. We talked for five minutes and I finally called the doctor. Later I heard that another twenty-four hours would have been too late, for the strep germ had already made great headway.

Ten o'clock. Two small boys stretched out on the floor, reading the funny books, oblivious of the cold by the door or the people who have to step over them.

Salesmen. Three in a row even on Saturday. Oh, well, they work, too, and all the best things I know, I have learned from salesmen. Money orders, coca colas, magazines, matches. A prescription to fill.

Telephone!

"Do you have green bath salts?" Hastily I scan the stock of salts,—Coty, Yardley,—Ah! Here is one,—

"Yes, Madam, we do carry green bath salts."

"Well, put them in the window to ripen." I felt as if I were running a slight temperature when I waited on the next customer. Pranksters on Saturday morning is too much!

"Baw! I dropped my penny down the magazine rack." One of the youthful readers seems to be in difficulty.

Another prescription. When it has been filled, "Don't look

like the same color to me as the last one." It is different. I tried to tell him that it was different, since the prescription called for different ingredients. But I know he feels he is going to die and it is a lifetime job to convince the average man that a woman has brains enough to be a druggist. I said brains, but it is not exactly what I mean; I mean patience and endurance.

Next, a flapper buying cosmetics! It's an education! A revelation! Though how such a conglomeration of colors could rest on one sweet heart-shaped face, is for an artist to answer.

Eleven o'clock. The girl who helps at the fountain comes on duty.

A hundred capsules to fill, a pint of emulsion, a dozen suppositories and a score of questions to answer.

"My mother wants to know if she can give aspirin to the baby, she has an earache?"

"My doctor told me to take three grains of thyroid a day and it makes me jumpy. What shall I do?"

"Could you take an hour off to sing at a funeral?" The last query came from a man who is a good customer and so was the man who died. So I called in a relief man, filled the next prescription to the tune of "Nearer My God to Thee" and left for the undertaking parlors.

Three o'clock. Out of a black dress and into a white uniform again.

Telephone!

"Send me a ten cent box of aspirin right away!" So the delivery goes with a ten cent item which costs twenty cents to deliver.

"Something for a cough."

Telephone,—

"I just scalded my arm. Send me something over quickly!" Only two miles away! The delivery is still on the aspirin truck!

"Will you cash this check for my mother?" Ten dollars! I looked at it and resisted the temptation to apply it on the account his mother had owed for two years.

Six o'clock. Precious hour! Time to eat. I make for the door, glancing furtively about to see if anyone dare detain me.

"Oh, Are you leaving? I just want to speak to you for a minute." It took ten minutes to listen and one to fill the order and once more I started for dinner.

Safely in the car. A neighbor spied me and demanded cough syrup—my cough syrup.

Next time I left by the back door. It's more complicated to unlock a double door, but at least I get my dinner.

Half an hour and I am back on the job again. Hastily I run a comb through my hair—apply a little lipstick—I might be asked to sell cosmetics and should be a fair example of what artificial application will do for a mere forty-year old. Back to waiting on customers.

Aspirin—cough syrup—soap—Kleenex—

"Will you see what I have in my eye?" I send her to a doctor.

A bottle of tablets for a customer who raves that he can buy them at Lawson's for half the price. I know he can't but I smilingly express my regret at being unable to meet the price. He takes the pills—he knows better, too.

Ten o'clock—ten thirty and time to close. Tired but happy! There's no monotony to this business of being a druggist.

Of the scores who pass through your door each day, some will like you and some dislike you. Some trust you with their lives, while a few will doubt that you have any grey matter at all. You will help many people. Very few will mention the fact, but at night when you turn the key in the door, there will be a warm, comfortable feeling of a day well spent.

Tomorrow is Sunday, and I lift my voice in song and I smile. But what the rector, the director and the little choir boys don't know is why I smile. For more than an hour I sleep. That is the secret between God and me.

―――❖―――

About the Author

Nellie Davis Poulsen was born in 1898 and raised in the Midlands of England. She was very close to her Irish Granny, and from her, she developed a keen interest in healing and the use of herbs. She worked in a hospital in Birmingham, England before and after World War I.

She came to America in 1923 with her daughter Ruth, and went directly to Royal Oak, Michigan where she soon worked in a pharmacy. She became a registered pharmacist, then opened her first drug store in 1929, and later owned five pharmacies. She received the National Hygia Award and has been entered in the *Who's Who of American Women* in the 1960's.

Many interests and talents enriched Nellie's life and that of her community. During all her years of hard work, she wrote two novels, *House of Sanctary* and *Hilltops Have Sunshine*. For 25 years she wrote articles for the *National Pharmaceutical Magazine*. She had a rich contralto voice with an English accent that found her singing on radio station WXYZ in Detroit, and in the choir at Christ Church, Cranbrook. Nellie established the public libraries in Atlanta, Hillman, and Lewiston and was an active board member for many years. She was also a key participant in the Atlanta Art Guild

Retirement gave her the opportunity to enjoy McCormick Lake and the beauty around her home in Atlanta, Michigan. She painted the seasons and views as she saw them. She wrote articles and book reviews for the *Montmorency County Tribune* for over thirty years.

At the age of 97, Nellie learned from her daughter Ruth of the plan to publish this book in response to many requests from her appreciative readers. Nellie was overjoyed at the prospect. Sadly her health failed rapidly thereafter and she died in October of 1995.

Living and Learning is a composite of Nellie Poulsen's newspaper columns and includes two true short stories written in the 30's. Her oil paintings have been photographed by her daughter Ruth Williams, who is a professional photographer, to illustrate some of the articles.

❖